The Little

Sport

Medicine

Series Editor: Daniel K. Onion

SECOND EDITION

Thomas M. Howard, MD
Program Director
VCU-Fairfax Family Practice Sports
Medicine Fellowship
Fairfax, Virginia

Janus D. Butcher, MD, FACSM
The Duluth Clinic
Department of Orthopedics
Duluth, Minnesota

JONES AND BARTLETT PUBLISHERS
Sudbury, Massachusetts
BOSTON   TORONTO   LONDON   SINGAPORE

World Headquarters

Jones and Bartlett
Publishers
40 Tall Pine Drive
Sudbury, MA 01776
978-443-5000
info@jbpub.com
www.jbpub.com

Jones and Bartlett
Publishers Canada
6339 Ormindale Way
Mississauga, ON L5V 1J2
CANADA

Jones and Bartlett
Publishers
International
Barb House, Barb Me
London W6 7PA
UK

Jones and Bartlett's books and products are available through most bookstores
and online booksellers. To contact Jones and Bartlett Publishers directly, call
800-832-0034, fax 978-443-8000, or visit our website www.jbpub.com.

Substantial discounts on bulk quantities of Jones and Bartlett's publications are avail
to corporations, professional associations, and other qualified organizations. For deta
and specific discount information, contact the special sales department at Jones and
Bartlett via the above contact information or send an email to specialsales@jbpub.c

Library of Congress Cataloging-in-Publication Data
Howard, Thomas M.
    The little black book of sports medicine / Thomas M. Howard and Janus D.
Butcher. — 2nd ed.
        p. ; cm.
    Rev. ed. of: Blackwell's primary care essentials. Sports medicine.
Blackwell Science, c2001.
    Includes bibliographical references and index.
    ISBN 0-7637-3865-4
    1. Sports medicine—Handbooks, manuals, etc.   2. Sports injuries—
Handbooks, manuals, etc.
    [DNLM: 1. Athletic Injuries—Handbooks.   2. Evidence-Based Medicine—
Handbooks.   3. Sports Medicine—Handbooks.   QT 29 H852L 2006]   I. Butcher,
Janus D.   II. Howard, Thomas M. Blackwell's primary care essentials.
Sports medicine.   III. Title.
RC1211.H69 2006
617.1′027—dc22

                                                                    2005019332

Production Credits
Executive Publisher: Christopher Davis
Production Director: Amy Rose
Associate Editor: Kathy Richardson
Production Assistant: Alison Meier
Associate Marketing Manager: Laura Kavigian
Manufacturing Buyer: Therese Connell

Composition: ATLIS Graphics
Cover Design: Anne Spencer
Cover Images: © Photos.com
Printing and Binding: Malloy, Inc.
Cover Printing: Malloy, Inc.

Printed in the United States of America
09   08   07   06   05   10   9   8   7   6   5   4   3   2   1

Contents

Chapter 14 The Foot   249

Cathy Fieseler, MD

Chapter 15 Neurology   267

Janus Butcher, MD

Chapter 16 Adolescent and Pediatric Problems   283

Diane Donnelly, MD,
Thomas Howard, MD, and
Harry McKinnon, MD

Chapter 17 Cardiovascular Problems   305

*Robert Oh, MD and
Charles Webb, MD*

Chapter 18 Issues Unique to the Female Athlete   325

Janus Butcher, MD

Chapter 19 Gastrointestinal Problems   333

Janus Butcher, MD

Chapter 20 Infectious Disease   343

Thomas Howard, MD

Chapter 21 Other Medical Problems   351

*Thomas Howard, MD and
Harry McKinnon, MD*

Chapter 22 Rehabilitation Exercises 365

Thomas Howard, MD and Gary Ho, MD

Preface

Every day primary care providers are challenged with occupational, recreational, and sports-induced injuries and medical problems. Nearly one-third of all office visits in the primary care setting are related to such problems. This problem-oriented book will help physicians (pediatricians, internists, and family physicians), nurse practitioners, and physician's assistants approach and deal with these issues more effectively.

The authors are grateful to the contributors for their expertise in this second edition of *The Little Black Book of Sports Medicine*.

Medical Abbreviations

5-HIAA	5-hydroxyindoleacetic acid	APGAR	Activity, Pulse, Grimace, Appearance, Respiration
AAA	Abdominal aortic aneurysm	APMHR	Age predicted maximum heart rate
AAS	Acute abdominal series	AR	Aldose reductase
AAT	Anterior apprehension test	ARDS	Adult respiratory distress syndrome
ABI	Ankle-brachial index	ASAP	As soon as possible
Abn	Abnormal	ASCVD	Arteriosclerotic cardiovascular disease
ABX	Antibiotics		
AC	Acromioclavicular	ASIS	Anterior superior iliac spine
AC OA	Acromioclavicular osteoarthritis	AST	Aspartate aminotransferase
ACE	Angiotensin converting enzyme	ATFL	Anterior Talofibular Ligament
ACL	Anterior cruciate ligament	ATL	Atypical lymphocytes
ACTH	Adrenocorticotropic hormone	ATP	Adenosine triphosphate
		AVN	Avascular necrosis
ADAMS	Aortic Dilation and Marfan's Syndrome	BAPS	Name of a balance board used in physical therapy
ADLs	Activities of daily living		
ADP	Adenosine diphosphate	BBB	Bundle branch block
AI	Aortic insufficiency	BCAA	Branch chain amino acids
AITFL	Anterior-Inferior Tibiofibular Ligament		
		bcp's	Birth control pills
aka	Also known as	BMI	Body Mass Index
ALT	Alanine aminotransferase	BP	Blood pressure
AM	Morning	BPD	Bipolar Disorder
AMS	Acute mountain sickness	BUN	Blood urea nitrogen
ANA	Antinuclear antibody	BW	Body weight
AP	Anterior-posterior		

CAD	Coronary artery disease	DMG	Dimethylglycine
CAM	"CAM" as in shape of a boot-type ankle/foot brace	DRE	Digital rectal exam
		DRUJ	Distal radial-ulnar joint
		DTR	Deep tendon reflex
CBC with Diff	Complete blood count with differential	DVT	Deep vein thrombosis
		EAA	Exercise-associated amenorrhea
CBC	Complete blood count		
CBT	Care body temperature	EAC	Exercise-associated collapse
CFL	Calacaneo-fibular Ligament	EBV	Epstein-Barr virus
		Echo	Echocardiogram
CHF	Congestive heart failure	ECR	Extensor carpi radialis
CMC	Carpal-metacarpal	ECRB	Extensor carpi radialis brevis
CP	Creatine phosphate		
CPK	Creatine phosphokinase	ECS	Exertional compartment syndrome
Cr	Creatinine		
CRP	C reactive protein	ECU	Extensor carpi ulnaris
CSF	Cerebrospinal fluid	EDC	Extensor digitorum communis
CT	Computed tomography		
CTS	Carpal tunnel syndrome	EDV	End diastolic volume
CV	Cardiovascular	EEG	Electroencephalogram
CVA	Cerebrovasular accident	EGD	Esophago-gastro-duodenoscopy
CVD	Cardiovascular disease		
CXR	Chest x-ray	EHL	Extensor halucus longus
		EKG	Electrocardiogram
DBL	Dreaded black line	EMG	Electromyogram
DEXA	Dual energy x-ray absorptiometry	EP	Electrophysiologic
		EPB	Extensor pollicis brevis
DF	Dorsiflexion	Epi	Epinephrine
DHEA	Dehydroepiandrosterone	EPO	Erythropoietin
DIC	Disseminated intravascular coagulation	ER	External rotators or external rotation
DIP	Distal interphalangeal joint	ESI	Epidural steroid injection
DISI	Dorsal intercalated segment instability	esp	Especially
		ESR	Erythrocyte sedimentation rate
DJD	Degenerative joint disease		
DM	Diabetes mellitus	ETOH	Ethanol

Ev	Eversion	HCM	Hypertrophic cardiomyopathy
eval	Evaluate	HDL	High-density lipoprotein
FABER	**F**lexion **AB**duction **E**xternal **R**otation	hep	Hepatitis
		HGH	Human growth hormone
FCU	Flexor carpi ulnaris	HIV	Human immunodeficiency virus
FD	Flexor digitorum		
FH	Family history	HNP	Herniated Nucleus Pulposis
FHL	Flexor Hallucis Longus		
FITT	**F**requency, **I**ntensity, **T**ime, **T**ype	HPA	Hypothalamic-pituitary axis
FSH	Follicle stimulating hormone	HR	Heart rate
		hr	Hour(s)
FSP	Fibrin split products	HRR	Heart rate reserve
FVC	Forced vital capacity	HS	At night
fx	Fracture	HTN	Hypertension
		hx	History
GABS	Group A beta-hemolytic Streptococcus	IBD	Inflammatory Bowel Disease
gc	Gonorrhea		
GGT	Gamma-glutamyl transpeptidase	IBS	Irritable bowel syndrome
		IBW	Ideal body weight
GH	Glenohumeral	ICB	Intracranial bleed
gi	Gastrointestinal	ICD	Implantable cardiac defibrillator
GI	Glycemic index		
GLDH	Glutamate dehydrogenase	IDT	Inferior dislocation test
GnRH	Gonadotropin releasing hormone	ie	In other words
		ILGF-1	Insulin-like growth factor
GXT	Graded exercise test	IM	Intramuscular
		Inf	Inferior
h/o	History of	IOC	International Olympic Committee
HACE	High Altitude Cerebral Edema		
		IOM	Interosseous membrane
HAPE	High Altitude Pulmonary Edema	IP	Interphalangeal
		IR	Internal rotation
HCG	Human chorionic gonadotropin	ITB	Iliotibial band
		iv	Intravenous

IVIG	Intravenous immunoglobulin	MTP	Metatarsal-phalangeal
		MTSS	Medial Tibial Stress Syndrome
JRA	Juvenile rheumatoid arthritis	MVA	Motor vehicle accident
		MVP	Mitral valve prolapse
kg	Kilogram	NCAA	National Collegiate Athletic Association
KOH	Potassium hydroxide		
		NCS	Nerve conduction study
LAT	Lateral	NCV	Nerve conduction velocities
LBM	Lean body mass		
LBP	Low back pain	NIH	National Institute of Health
LCL	Lateral collateral ligament		
LCP	Legg-Calvé-Perthes	NSAID	Non-steroidal anti-inflammatory drug
LDH	Lactate dehydrogenase		
LDL	Low-density lipoproteins		
LE	Lower extremity	O2	Oxygen
LES	Lower esophageal sphincter	OA	Osteoarthritis
		OCD	Osteochondral defect or Osteochondritis Dessicans
LFT's	Liver function tests		
LH	Luteinizing hormone	OCL	Osteocohondral lesion
LQTS	Long QT Syndrome	OMT	Osteopathic manipulative therapy
LT	Luno-triquetral		
		ORIF	Operative reduction and internal fixation
MB	Myocardial band		
MC	Metacarpal	OTC	Over-the-counter
MCL	Medical collateral ligament		
		PA	Posterior-anterior
MCP	Metacarpal-phalangeal joint(s)	PCL	Posterior cruciate ligament
		pCO2	Partial pressure of carbon dioxide
MI	Myocardial infarction; or mitral insufficiency		
		PDT	Posterior dislocation test
min	Minute(s)	PE	Pulmonary embolism
MO	Myositis Ossificans Mod	PF	Plantarflexion or palmer flexion
MR	Mitral regurgitation		
MRI	Magnetic resonance imaging	PIN	Posterior Interosseous Nerve

PIP	Proximal interphalangeal joint	ROM	Range of motion
PIPJ	PIP joint	RPPS	Retropatellar pain syndrome
PITFL	Posterior-inferior Tibiofibular Ligament	RSD/ CRPS	Reflex Sympathetic Dystrophy/Complex Regional Pain Syndrome
PMN	Polymorphonuclear neutrophils		
PPA	Phenylpropanolamine	RV	Right ventricle
PPE	Preparticipation physical exam	RVH	Right ventricular hypertrophy
PRIC- EMM	Protect, rest, ice, compression, elevation, medications, modalities	SAH	Subarachnoid hemorrhage
		SBE	Subacute bacterial endocarditis
PSA	Prostate specific antigen	SCFE	Slipped Capital Femoral Epiphysis
PT	Physical therapy		
pt(s)	Patient(s)	secs	Seconds
PTFL	Posterior talofibular ligaments	SI	Sacroiliac
		SITS	**S**upraspinatus, **I**nfraspinatus, **T**eres Minor, **S**ubscapularis
PUD	Peptic ulcer disease		
Q2H	Every 2 hours		
qd	Daily	SL	Scapholunate
QID	4 times a day	SLAP	Superior Labral Anterior-Posterior
QT	QT interval of QRS complex		
		SLJ	Sinding-Larsen-Johanssen
		SLR	Straight-leg raise
r/o	Rule out	SPECT	Single-photon emission computed tomography
RA	Rheumatoid arthritis		
rbc	Red blood cell	SQ	Subcutaneous
RC	Rotator cuff	SS	Supraspinatus
RDA	Recommended daily allowance	SSRI	Selective serotonin reuptake inhibitor
rEPO	Recombinant erythropoietin	STD	Sexually transmitted disease
RF	Rheumatoid factor	SV	Stroke volume
RICE	Rest, Ice, Compression, Elevation		
		TCA	Tricyclic antidepressant

TENS	Transcutaneous electrical nerve stimulation	VMA	Vanillylmandelic acid
TFCC	Triangular fibrocartilage complex	VMO	Vastus medialis obliqus
		VO$_2$max	Maximal oxygen consumption
TIA	Transient ischemic attack	VO$_2$R	Reserve oxygen
TID	Three times a day		consumption
TLSO	Thoraco-lumbar spinal orthosis	w/o	Without
TM	Tympanic membrane	WBC	White blood cells or white
TMJ	Temporal mandibular joint		blood count
TSH	Thyroid stimulating hormone	wk	Week(s)
TTP	Tenderness to palpation	XC	Cross-country
		XR	Xray
UA	Urinalysis		
UCL	Ulnar collateral ligament	y/o	Years old
UE	Upper extremity		
UTI	Urinary tract infection	α-KIC	Alpha-ketoisocaporate
		β-HMB	Beta-hydroxy-methylbutyrate
VISI	Volar intercalated segment instability		

Journal and Reference Abbreviations

AAOS Instr Course Lect	American Academy of Orthopedic Surgery Instruction Course Lectures
Acta Orthop Scand	Acta Orthopedia Scandinavia
Adol Med	Adolescent Medicine
Adv Stud Med	Advanced Studies in Medicine
AHCPR	Agency for Health Care Policy and Research
Am Fam Phys	American Family Physician
Am J Gastroenterol	American Journal of Gastroenterology
Am J Knee Surg	American Journal of Knee Surgery
Am J Orthop	American Journal of Orthopedics
Am J Phys Med Rehabil	American Journal of Physical Medicine and Rehabilitation
Am J Sports Med	American Journal of Sports Medicine
Amer J Clin Nutrition	American Journal of Clinical Nutrition
Ankle	Ankle
Ann EM	Annals of Emergency Medicine
Ann IM	Annals of Internal Medicine
Ann Pharm	Annals of Pharmacotherapy
Arch Fam Med	Archives of Family Medicine
Arch IM	Archives of Internal Medicine
Aust J Sci Med Sport	Australian Journal of Science and Medicine in Sport
Aust J Sci Med	Australia Journal of Science Medicine
Aviat Space Environ Med	Aviation Space and Environmental Medicine

Br J Clin Pharm	British Journal of Clinical Pharmacology
Br J Sports Medicine	British Journal of Sports Medicine
Cardio Clin	Cardiology Clinics
Cardiol Rev	Cardiology in Review
Clin Anat	Clinical Anatomy
Clin Auton Res	Clinical Autonomic Research
Clin Dermatol	Clinics in Dermatology
Clin Fam Practice	Clinic in Family Practice
Clin J Sp Med	Clinical Journal of Sports Medicine
Clin Orthop Relat Res	Clinical Orthopedics and Related Research
Clin Orthop	Clinical Orthopedics
Clin Podiatr Med Surg	Clinics in Podiatric Medicine and Surgery
Clin Sports Med	Clinics in Sports Medicine
CPEM	Clinical Pediatric Emergency Medicine
Crit Care Clin	Critical Care Clinics
Curr Opin Orthop	Current Opinions in Orthopaedics
Curr Opin Rheumatol	Current Opinions in Rheumatology
Curr Sports Med Rep	Current Sports Medicine Reports
Dig Dis Sci	Digestive Disease Science
Dis Mon	Disease-a-Month
Emerg Med Clin N Am	Emergency Medical Clinics of North America
Eur J Appl Physiol	European Journal of Applied Physiology
Exerc Sport Sci Rev	Exercise and Sport Sciences Reviews
Fed Pract	Federal Practitioner

Foot Ankle Int	Foot and Ankle International
Gastroenterol Clin No Amer	Gastroenterology Clinic of North America
Geriatrics	Geriatrics
GSSI Sports Sci Ex	Gatorade Sports Science Institute Sports Science Exchange
Hand Clin	Hand Clinics
Immunol Aller Clin N Am	Immunology and Allergy Clinics of North America
Int J Biosoc Med Res	International Journal of Biosocial and Medical Research
Int J Sp Nutr	International Journal of Sports Nutrition
Int J Sports Med	International Journal of Sports Medicine
J Accid Emerg Med	Journal of Accident and Emergency Medicine
J Allergy Clin Immun	Journal of Allergy and Clinical Immunology
J Am Acad Dermatol	Journal of the American Academy of Dermatology
J Am Acad Orthop Sug	Journal of the American Academy of Orthopedic Surgery
J Am Board Fam Prac	Journal of the American Board of Family Practice
J Am Coll Cardiol	Journal of the American College of Cardiology
J Anat	Journal of Anatomy
J Appl Physiol	Journal of Applied Physiology
J Bone Joint Surg	Journal of Bone and Joint Surgery
J Clin Endo and Met	Journal of Clinical Endocrinology and Metabolism
J Emerg Med	Journal of Emergency Medicine
J Hand Surg	Journal of Hand Surgery

J Nutr	Journal of Nutrition
J of All and Clin Imm	Journal of Allergy and Clinical Immunology
J Reprod Med	Journal of Reproductive Medicine
J Rheumatol	Journal of Rheumatology
J Sport Sci	Journal of Sports Sciences
J Trauma	Journal of Trauma
Jama	Journal of the American Medical Association
Lancet	Lancet
Major Probl Clin Pediatr	Major Problems in Clinical Pediatrics
Manual Sports Med	Safran MR, VanCamp SD, McKeak DB, eds. LWW, July 1998
Mayo Clin Proc	Mayo Clinical Proceedings
Med Clin N Amer	Medical Clinics of North America
Med Sci Sports Exerc	Medicine and Science in Sports and Exercise
Mil Med	Military MedicineN Z Med New Zealand Journal of Medicine
Nejm	New England Journal of Medicine
Neurol Clin	Neurology Clinics
Neurol	Neurology
Nut Aspects of Ex	Nutritional Aspects of Exercise
Nutrition	Nutrition
Ortho Clin North Am	Orthopedic Clinics of North America
Orthop Rev	Orthopedic Reviews
Orthopedic Sports Med	*Orthopedic Sports Medicine* DeLee JC and Drez D, eds. WB Saunders, Philadelphia, 2003

Orthopedics	Orthopedics
Pain Prac	Pain Practice
Ped Clin North Am	Pediatric Clinics of North America
Ped Rv	Pediatric Review
Pediatr Radiol	Pediatric Radiology
Peds	Pediatrics
Phy Sportsmed	The Physician and Sportsmedicine
Phys Med Rehabil Clin N Am	Physical Medicine and Rehabilitation Clinics of North America
Prim Care	Primary Care: Clinics in Office Practice
Respirology	Respirology
Rheum Disease Clin N Am	Rheumatic Disease Clinics of North America
Science	Science
Semin Arthroplasty	Seminars in Arthroplasty
Skeletal Radiol	Skeletal Radiology
South Med J	Southern Medical Journal
South Med	Southern Medicine
Spine	Spine
Sports Med Arthro Rev	Sports Medicine & Arthroscopy Review
Sports Med	Sports Medicine
Stroke	Stroke
Surg Clin North Amer	Surgical Clinics of North America
Tech Hand Up Extrem Surg	Techniques in Hand and Upper Extremity Surgery
Urol Clin N Am	Urology Clinic of North America

Contributors

Janus D. Butcher, MD, FACSM
The Duluth Clinic
Department of Orthopedics
Duluth, MN

Thomas M. Howard, MD
Program Director
Sports Medicine Fellowship
VCU-Fairfax Family Practice
Fairfax, VA

Sean Mulvaney, MD
MAJ, MC, USA
Stuttgart, GE

Francis G. O'Connor, MD
COL, MC, USA
Chief, Family Medicine
Associate Program Director
NCC, Primary Care Sports Medicine
   Fellowship
DeWitt Army Community
   Hospital
Ft Belvoir, VA

Cathy Fieseler, MD
Director of Sports Medicine
Trinity Mother Frances Health
   System
Tyler, TX

Harry McKinnon, MD
LTC, MC, USA
DeWitt Army Community Hospital
Ft Belvoir, VA

Robert Oh, MD
MAJ, MC, USA
Madigan Army Medical Center
Ft Lewis, WA

Koji Nishimura, MD
COL, MC, USA
Commander,
Basset Army Hospital
Fort Wainwright, AK

Wade Lillegard, MD
The Duluth Clinic
Duluth, MN

John Glorioso, MD
LTC, MC, USA
Tripler Army Medical Center
Honolulu, HI

Paul Pasquina, MD
LTC, MC, USA
Program Director
NCC Consortium, PM&R Residency
Walter Reed Army Medical Center
Washington, DC

Charles Webb, MD
MAJ, MC, USA
Martin Army Community Hospital
Ft Benning, GA

Neil Johnson, MD
LTC, MC, USA
Munson Army Health Center
Ft Leavenworth, KS

Ted Epperley, MD
Chairman and Program Director
Family Practice Residency of Idaho
Boise, Idaho

Brian Unwin, MD
LTC, MC, USA
Department of Family Medicine
USUHS School of Medicine
Bethesda, MD

Gary Ho, MD
VCU-Fairfax Family Practice
Fairfax, VA

Diane Donnelly, MD
VCU-Fairfax Family Practice
Fairfax, VA

Notice

We have made every attempt to summarize accurately and concisely a multitude of references. However the reader is reminded that times and medical knowledge change, transcription or understanding error is always possible, and crucial details are omitted whenever such a comprehensive distillation as this is attempted in limited space. And the primary purpose of this compilation is to cite literature on various sides of controversial issues; knowing where "truth" lies is usually difficult. We cannot, therefore, guarantee that every bit of information is absolutely accurate or complete. The reader should affirm that cited recommendations are reasonable still, by reading the original articles and checking other sources, including local consultants as well as recent literature, before applying them.

Drugs and medical devices are discussed that may have limited availability controlled by the Food and Drug Administration (FDA) for use only in research study or clinical trial. The drug information presented has been derived from reference sources, recently published data, and pharmaceutical tests. Research, clinical practice, and government regulations often change the accepted standard in this field. When consideration is being given to use of any drug in the clinical setting, the clinician or reader is responsible for determining FDA status of the drug, reading the package insert, and prescribing information for the most up-to-date recommendations on dose, precautions, and contraindications and determining the appropriate usage for the product. This is especially important in the case of drugs that are new or seldom used.

Chapter 1

Injections

1.1 General Principles

Clin Sports Med 1995;14:353; Geriatrics 1990;45:45; Curr Opin
   Rheumatol 1999;11:417

Medications:
- Dexamethasone acetate (Decadron LA) 8 mg/cc
- Triamcinolone diacetate (Aristocort) 40 mg/cc
- Local anesthetics: lidocaine 1%, bupivacaine 0.25%

Mode of Action/Effects:
- Inhibits release of prostaglandin synthesis, cytokines, and
  chemical mediators.
- Inhibit activation and function of neutrophils, macrophages,
  fibroblasts, and basophils.

General Side Effects/Complications:
- Local effects and complications: infection (very low risk with
  proper technique), nerve injury, pneumothorax, subcutaneous
  fat atrophy, skin color changes.
- Allergic reactions: anesthetic or corticosteroid preparation.
- Tendon and joint complications: tendon rupture, articular car-
  tilage damage, osteoporosis.
- Other reactions: steroid flare (2% of injections), vasovagal
  response (most common with upper extremity injections).
- Diabetes mellitus: hyperglycemia.
- Glaucoma: Reported potential complication. Rare in practice.

Contraindications:
- Acute systemic infection, joint infection, or cellulitis at injection site.
- Poorly controlled diabetes.
- History of reaction to any components of injection solution.
- Injection into a prosthetic joint or fracture site.

1.2 de Quervain's Tenosynovitis

Indication:
- Reduce pain in extensor pollicis brevis and abductor pollicis to allow adequate rehabilitation and tissue healing.

Anatomy:
- EPB and abductor pollicis tendons contained in 1st dorsal wrist compartment.
- Tendons form the dorsal and volar boundaries of the anatomic snuffbox.

Procedure:
- 25-gauge, 1½-inch needle is inserted at the anatomic snuffbox into the 1st dorsal wrist compartment directed proximally (Figure 1.1).

Medication:
- 1-2 cc dexamethasone acetate (Decadron LA) 8 mg/cc in 3 cc of lidocaine (1%).
- 1-2 cc triamcinolone (40 mg/cc) in 3 cc of lidocaine (1%).

Precautions:
- Avoid injection into subcutaneous fat (may cause fat atrophy).
- Superficial injection may cause skin discoloration.

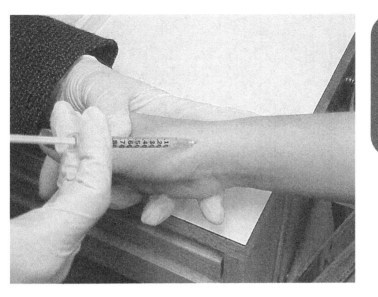

Figure 1.1   de Quervain's Tenosynovitis Injection

1.3   Trigger Finger

Indication:

- Painful catching or locking of finger with active flexion.

Anatomy:

- Flexor tendon nodule typically just proximal to MCP joint.
- Will translate with active flexion/extension of the affected digit.

Procedure:

- Using a ⅝-inch, 25-gauge instill solution into flexor tendon sheath at the palpable nodule (Figure 1.2).

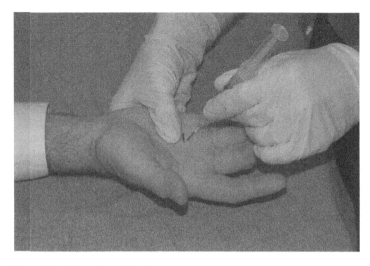

Figure 1.2   Trigger Finger Injection

Medication:
- 3/4 cc dexamethasone acetate (Decadron LA) 8 mg/cc in 3 cc of lidocaine (1%).
- 3/4 cc triamcinolone (40 mg/cc) in 1/4 cc of lidocaine (1%).

Precautions:
- Ensure that pain is not the result of infectious flexor tenosynovitis.
- Avoid injection into subcutaneous fat (may cause fat atrophy).

1.4   Extensor Carpi Ulnaris

Indication:
- Ulnar wrist pain related to inflammation of the ECU tendon.

Anatomy:
- ECU tendon palpable at distal ulna with swelling in the sheath often appreciated several cm proximal from this point.

Procedure:
- Medial wrist at the distal ulna is sterilely prepared and a 1½-inch, 25-gauge needle is inserted at the distal ulna directed proximally. Solution should be palpable as it fills the ECU sheath (Figure 1.3).

Medication:
- 1-2 cc dexamethasone acetate (Decadron LA) 8 mg/cc in 3 cc of lidocaine (1%).
- 1-2 cc triamcinolone (40 mg/cc) in 3 cc of lidocaine (1%).

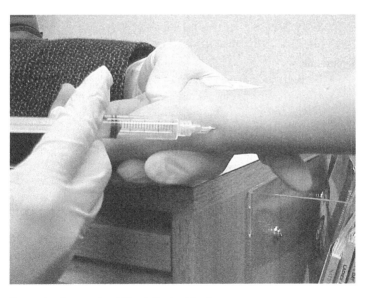

Figure 1.3 Extensor Carpi Ulnaris Tendon injection

Precautions:
- Avoid injection into subcutaneous fat (may cause fat atrophy).
- Superficial injection may cause skin discoloration.

1.5   Triangular Fibrocartilage Complex

Indication:
- Chronic ulnar-sided wrist pain due to tear or degeneration of the TFCC.

Anatomy:
- TFCC fills the space between the distal ulna (ulnar styloid) and proximal medial carpus.

Procedure:
- After sterile prep, solution is injected through a 1½-inch, 25-gauge needle via a medial approach. The needle is inserted just distal to the ulnar styloid (Figure 1.4).

Medication:
- 1-2 cc triamcinolone (40 mg/cc) in 3 cc of lidocaine (1%).
- 1-2 cc dexamethasone acetate (Decadron LA) 8 mg/cc in 3 cc of lidocaine (1%).

Precautions:
- Avoid injection into subcutaneous fat (may cause fat atrophy).
- Superficial injection may cause skin discoloration.

1.6   Carpal Tunnel Syndrome

Indication:
- Reduction of flexor tendon inflammation to reduce pain and median nerve compression.

Anatomy:
- Carpal tunnel formed by the proximal carpal row and flexor retinaculum.

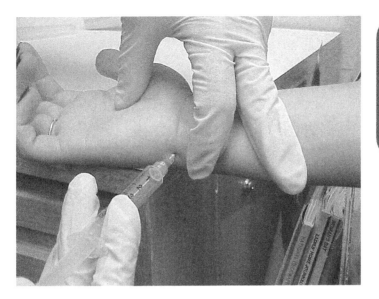

Figure 1.4 TFCC Injection

- Contains flexor digitorum profundus and superficialis, flexor policis longus, flexor carpi radialis, and the median nerve.

Procedure:
- After sterile preparation, a 25-gauge needle is placed beneath the flexor retinaculum at the radial border of the palmaris longus at the distal flexor crease. The needle is directed at an approximate 45° angle proximally (Figure 1.5).

Medication:
- 1 cc triamcinolone (40 mg/cc) in 1 cc of lidocaine (1%).

Precautions:
- Avoid injection into subcutaneous fat (may cause fat atrophy).
- Superficial injection may cause skin discoloration.

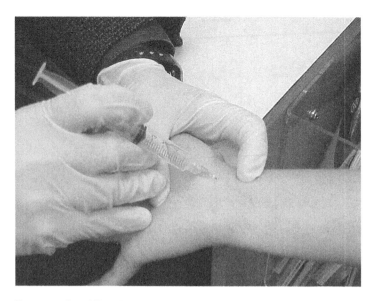

Figure 1.5 Carpal Tunnel Injection

- Avoid injection into the median nerve (patient will complain of shooting pain into hand).
- Relapse of symptoms is very common within 1 month of injection.

1.7 Tennis Elbow

Indication:
- Tenderness at origin of ECRB tendon on lateral epicondyle.

Anatomy:
- Common extensor tendon (extensor carpi radialis brevis, extensor digitorum, extensor digiti minimi, extensor carpi ulnaris) origin at the lateral epicondyle.

Procedure:

- After sterile preparation, solution is injected in a wide pattern along the insertion of the extensor tendons (Figure 1.6).

Medication:

- 1-2 cc triamcinolone (40 mg/cc) in 3 cc of lidocaine (1%).
- 1-2 cc dexamethasone acetate (Decadron LA) 8 mg/cc in 3 cc of lidocaine (1%).

Precautions:

- Avoid injection into subcutaneous fat (may cause fat atrophy).
- Superficial injection may cause skin discoloration.

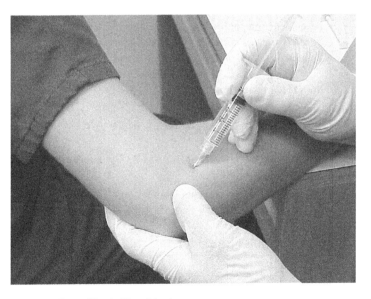

Figure 1.6 Lateral Tennis Elbow Injection

1.8 Subacromial Space

Indication:
- Reduction of pain due to inflammation of supraspinatus tendon, subacromial bursa, or lateral impingement.

Anatomy:
- Subacromial space formed by acromial arch (acromion and coracoacromial ligament) superiolaterally, supraspinatus muscle inferiorly, clavicle anteriorly, and the spine of the scapula posteriorly.
- Potential space occupied by subacromial bursa.

Procedure:
- After sterile preparation, 1½-inch, 25-gauge needle is introduced at the posteriolateral shoulder (junction of the posterior and middle deltoid muscle), just below the acromion. Needle should be parallel to the floor and directed toward the AC joint (Figure 1.7).

Medication:
- 1-2 cc dexamethasone acetate (Decadron LA) 8 mg/cc in 3 cc of lidocaine (1%).
- 1-2 cc triamcinolone (40 mg/cc) in 7-8 cc of lidocaine (1%).

Precautions:
- Avoid injection into subcutaneous fat (may cause fat atrophy).
- Superficial injection may cause skin discoloration.

1.9 Intra-Articular Shoulder

Indication:
- Relief of pain associated with osteoarthritis, undersurface supraspinatus tendinitis/partial thickness tear, or adhesive capsulitis.

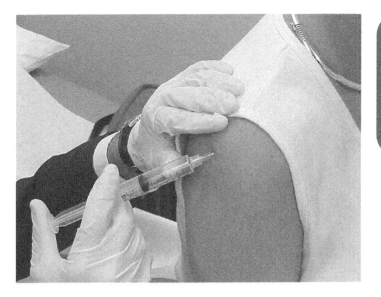

Figure 1.7 Shoulder Subacromial Space Injection

Anatomy:
- Capsule of glenohumeral joint lies just deep to the coracoid process from an anterior approach.

Procedure:
- After sterile preparation, 1½-inch, 25-gauge needle is introduced 1 cm lateral and 1 cm inferior to the coracoid. Gentle passive internal rotation of the shoulder after placement of the needle will confirm location by causing paradoxical motion of the needle (Figure 1.8).

Medication:
- 1-2 cc dexamethasone acetate (Decadron LA) 8 mg/cc in 3 cc of lidocaine (1%).
- 1-2 cc triamcinolone (40 mg/cc) in 7-8 cc of lidocaine (1%).

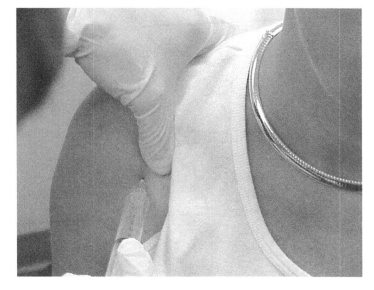

Figure 1.8 Intra-Articular Shoulder

Precautions:
- Anatomic landmarks must be assured to avoid placement of the needle too far medially (risk of pneumothorax), or inferiorly (risk of vascular or neurologic injury).

1.10 Acromioclavicular Joint

Indication:
- Relief of pain related to AC arthritis, osteolysis, and subacute AC separation.

Anatomy:
- The AC is typically angled at an approximate 45° angle directed midline caudally. The capsule lies just below the subcutaneous tissue.

Procedure:

- After sterile preparation, a 1½-inch, 25-gauge needle is inserted at the superior-lateral AC joint directed inferior-medially. May be difficult with significant DJD. It is often helpful to view the patient's radiograph while inserting the needle (Figure 1.9).

Medication:

- 1-2 cc dexamethasone acetate (Decadron LA) 8 mg/cc in 3 cc of lidocaine (1%).
- 1-2 cc triamcinolone (40 mg/cc) in 2-3 cc of lidocaine (1%).

Precautions:

- To ensure appropriate placement in AC joint, aspirate after injection. This will return some medication to syringe and confirm proper placement.

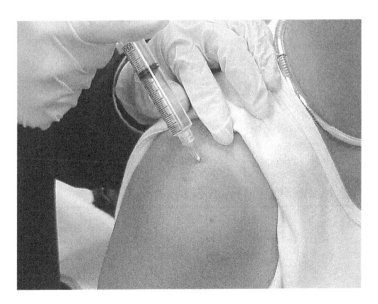

Figure 1.9 Acromioclavicular Joint Injection

1.11 Trochanteric Bursitis

Indication:
- Pain relief to allow participation in physical therapy, exercise, and continued activities of daily living.

Anatomy:
- Up to three separate bursae along the superior margin of the greater trochanter. Are found between the ITB and trochanter.

Procedure:
- After sterile preparation, palpate the soft tissue at the superior margin of the trochanter to identify the points of maximal tenderness. Insert a 2″ or longer, 25-gauge needle and inject solution as the needle is withdrawn. The bursa is irritated transiently by the anesthetic and will reproduce the patient's symptoms. The remainder of the solution is injected at this point (Figure 1.10).

Medication:
- 2-3 cc dexamethasone acetate (Decadron LA) 8 mg/cc in 10 cc of lidocaine (1%).
- 2-3 cc triamcinolone (40 mg/cc) in 10 cc of lidocaine (1%).

Precautions:
- Sciatic nerve lies deep and posterior to the trochanter.
- If bony contact is made (femoral neck), the injection will be intra-articular.

1.12 Iliotibial Band Friction Syndrome

Indication:
- Relief of pain related to acute or chronic irritation of ITB as it crosses the lateral femoral condyle.

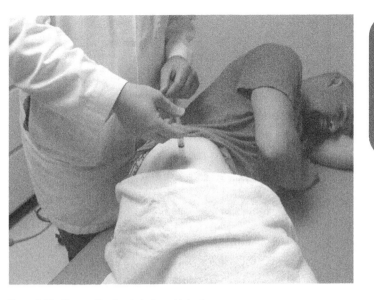

Figure 1.10 Greater Trochanteric Bursal Injection

Anatomy:
- The iliotibial band (ITB) arises from the tensor fascialata muscle in the lateral buttocks and runs along the lateral leg to its insertion at Gerdy tubercle on the anteriolateral tibia.
- Irritation typically occurs at contact with lateral femoral condyle (Figure 1.11).

Procedure:
- The point of maximal tenderness is identified and area is prepped in a sterile fashion. A 25-gauge needle is inserted and the solution injected beneath the ITB in a wide area.

Medication:
- 1-2 cc dexamethasone acetate (Decadron LA) 8 mg/cc in 3 cc of lidocaine (1%).
- 1-2 cc triamcinolone (40 mg/cc) in 3 cc of lidocaine (1%).

1.12   Iliotibial Band Friction Syndrome   **15**

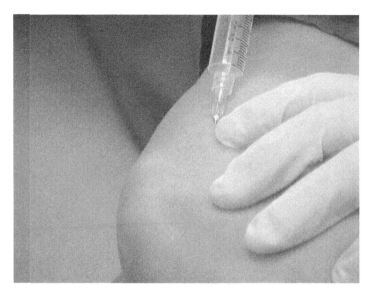

Figure 1.11   Iliotibial Band Friction Syndrome Injection

Precautions:
- Avoid injection into subcutaneous fat (may cause fat atrophy).
- Superficial injection may cause skin discoloration.

1.13 Intra-Articular Knee

Indication:
- Relief of pain due to degenerative joint disease, subacute meniscal tear or PFD.

Anatomy:
- Joint formed by articulation of tibia, femur, and patella. Continuous space from suprapatellar pouch to patellar tendon insertion.

Procedure:

- Multiple approaches possible. Knee should be thoroughly prepped with betadine and sterile techniques employed.
- Anterior approach: With the patient sitting and the knee flexed 90° a 1½-inch, 25-gauge needle is inserted on either the lateral or medial border of the patellar tendon. The needle is directed directly into the notch and the solution is injected into the notch (Figure 1.12).
- Lateral suprapatellar approach: With patient supine, the superior-lateral margin of the patella is palpated and a 25-gauge needle is inserted below the patella. The solution is instilled at this point. This approach is also used for aspiration. A 22-gauge needle is inserted in a similar fashion. Aspiration is accomplished with a 60-cc syringe. The aspiration syringe may

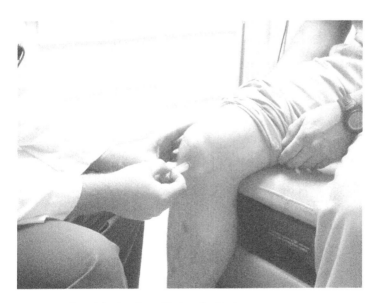

Figure 1.12 Knee Injection, Seated Peripatellar Tendon

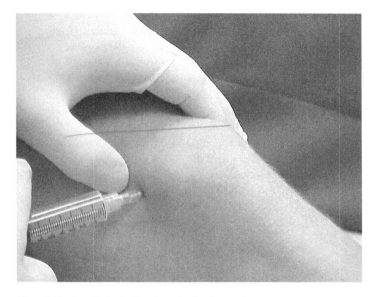

Figure 1.13 Intra-Articular Knee Injection/Aspiration, Supine

then be replaced with the syringe containing the steroid solution and the injection accomplished through the same needle (Figure 1.13).

Medication:
- 1-2 cc dexamethasone acetate (Decadron LA) 8 mg/cc in 3 cc of lidocaine (1%).
- 1-2 cc triamcinolone (40 mg/cc) in 7-8 cc of lidocaine (1%).

Precautions:
- Avoid injection into the ACL as this is quite painful.
- Limit injections to 2 to 3 injections in 12-month period. Repetitive injection can lead to softening of cartilage and further damage.

- Avoid injection into subcutaneous fat (may cause fat atrophy).
- Superficial injection may cause skin discoloration.

1.14 Plantar Fascia

Indication:
- Relief of pain due to inflammation of the plantar fascia origin.

Anatomy:
- Plantar fascia originates at the anterior plantar calcaneous and fans out at its distal insertion on the midmetatarsals. This structure forms the medial longitudinal arch (in part).

Procedure:
- Medial approach is significantly less painful than the plantar approach.
- Prep skin sterilely. Patient actively dorsiflexes the foot and great toe which will accentuate the medial margin of the plantar fascia.
- Palpate the anterior calcaneous and insert a 1½-inch, 25-gauge needle superior to the plantar fascia. Spread the medication in a fan-like pattern at the origin of the fascia (Figure 1.14).

Medication:
- 1-2 cc dexamethasone acetate (Decadron LA) 8 mg/cc in 3 cc of lidocaine (1%).
- 1-2 cc triamcinolone (40 mg/cc) in 3 cc of lidocaine (1%).

Precautions:
- Avoid injection into the heel fat pad (may cause fat atrophy).
- Superficial injection may cause skin discoloration.
- Avoid median plantar nerve.

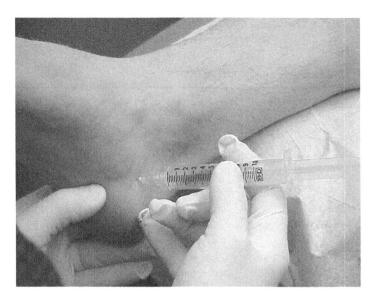

Figure 1.14 Plantar Fascia Injection

Chapter 2

Environmental Injuries

2.1 Acute Mountain Sickness

Respirology 2004;9:485; Br J Sports Med 1999;33:376

Cause: Hypoxia associated with rapid ascent to altitude.

Epidem:
- Altitude illness develops at elevations above 2,000-2,400 m, the elevation of most ski resorts in the western United States.
- Of lowland residents visiting these altitudes, approximately 25% develop acute mountain sickness.
- Up to 54% of people traveling abruptly to altitudes above 4,000 meters develop AMS.
- 20% of experienced climbers develop symptoms of AMS.
- Others at risk include balloon riders, campers, and passengers in unpressurized aircraft (eg, parachutists).
- Children more susceptible than adults.
- Alcohol consumption, smoking, and rigorous exercise upon arrival to altitude predispose to AMS.

Pathophys:
- Oxygen saturation drops below 90% at 2,500 m in most people.
- Hypoxia leads to low arterial oxygenation in cerebral blood flow, which leads to hyperventilation and respiratory alkalosis.
- Sodium retention resulting from hypoxia to the sodium pump leads to fluid retention.

- Rapid ascent does not allow the body to acclimate to these changes.

Sx:

- Throbbing headache, malaise, lethargy, anorexia, sleep disturbances, nausea, vomiting, and a dry cough or mild dyspnea.
- Typically develop within 8-24 hr of ascent and resolve without specific treatment in 24-72 hr.

Si:

- Tachycardia.
- Peripheral fluid retention (edema).

Crs:

- Generally benign, self-limited condition that resolves without sequelae.
- Failure to improve within 24-48 hr and/or the development of pulmonary or neurologic symptoms may indicate the development of high-altitude cerebral edema (HACE) or high-altitude pulmonary edema (HAPE).

Lab:

- None; however, other causes of AMS symptoms should be entertained (toxins, hypoglycemia, meningitis, etc).

Rx:

- Stop the ascent and rest or plan acclimatization day in air travel to altitude.
- Avoid alcohol and vigorous exercise early at altitude. Moderate exercise assists with acclimatization.
- Acetaminophen or ibuprofen may help alleviate the headache.
- Antiemetics may help alleviate the nausea.
- Acetazolamide (Diamox) 250 mg tid is a carbonic anhydrase inhibitor that stimulates ventilation and can improve the symptoms of AMS:
  1. In more severe cases or in those allergic to sulfas, dexamethasone (Decadron) 2-4 mg every 6 hr followed by a taper, may be used.

- Descent from altitude, oxygen therapy, and hyperbaric treatment are generally not necessary for AMS.

2.2 High-Altitude Cerebral Edema (HACE) and High-Altitude Pulmonary Edema (HAPE)

Stroke 2005;36:557; Ann IM 2005;142:591; Med Sci Sports Exerc 1994;26:195; Crit Care Clin 1999;15:265

Cause:
- High-altitude cerebral edema (HACE) is associated with rising intracranial pressure brought on by an alteration of dynamic autoregulation of cerebral blood flow. This results in overperfusion of capillaries and vasogenic cerebral edema.
- High-altitude pulmonary edema (HAPE) is caused by exaggerated pulmonary hypertension and high capillary pressure inducing a high permeability-type lung edema.

Epidem:
- Risk factors include: elevation attained, speed of ascent, and a history of previous HAPE. Strenuous exercise performed immediately upon arrival to altitude may also contribute.
- The reported incidence ranges from 0.01-15.5% of those ascending to high altitude.
- Mortality of HACE approaches 60% if coma ensues.
- A genetic predisposition may exist.

Pathophys:
- The mechanism of injury in HACE is not well understood, but is probably related to hypoxic cerebral vasodilation.
- Sympathetic vasoconstrictor overactivity and endothelial dysfunction (impaired nitric oxide release and augmented endothelial-1 release) may contribute to pulmonary hypertension in HAPE-prone individuals.
  1. Hypoxic pulmonary vasoconstriction leads to hyperperfusion and alveolar flooding.

2. The discrepancy between perfusion and ventilation in portions of the lung is the most likely pathophysiology in HAPE.
3. Other mechanisms may also contribute to HAPE including sympathetic nervous system discharge from cerebral vasodilation.

Sx:

- Symptoms of AMS are present with all forms of altitude injury and include headache, nausea, vomiting, anorexia, lightheadedness, dizziness, and are worsened by exertion.
- Typical symptoms of HACE include: unrelenting headache associated with vomiting, truncal ataxia, impaired mental status (confusion, poor judgment, delirium), and severe lassitude. Hemiparesis, hemiplegia, seizures, and coma are less common but suggest progression of this syndrome. HACE can develop within 24 hr of AMS, but typically will be delayed 1-3 d.
- HAPE symptoms are mostly respiratory and include dyspnea, cough, fatigue, chest pain, weakness, and lethargy. Cough may be frothy or blood stained as a result of capillary distension and leakage.

Si:

- Patients developing HACE may show nonspecific neurologic deficits (ranging from ataxia to coma) in addition to the signs of AMS (tachycardia, generalized edema).
- HAPE patients can show tachypnea, orthopnea, tachycardia, low-grade fever, and cyanosis.
- Lung auscultation may reveal rales, but the degree of crackles may not reflect the severity of pulmonary compromise.

Crs:

- While AMS is a generally benign, self-limiting condition that improves with acclimatization, HACE and HAPE are very dangerous clinical syndromes requiring prompt treatment as pulmonary failure and death may occur within hr of symptom onset.

- Symptoms of HACE or HAPE can resolve within a few days if immediate descent and treatment have occurred.
- Previous episodes increase the risk for future recurrence.
- Prevention is important:
  1. Ascend no more than 2,000 m/d.
  2. Maximize physical conditioning and climbing experience before entering high altitude environments.
  3. Avoid dehydration, medications, alcohol, and tobacco.

Lab:

- Arterial blood gas (if available) may demonstrate hypoxia and may be useful to show improvement with therapy.
- Other causes of altered mental status and cardiopulmonary disease should be ruled out with any means necessary (chemistry, CSF, CBC).

Other Testing:

- Chest radiograph may be normal or appear as mild congestive heart failure.

Rx:

- Descent from altitude is key.
- Oxygen (2-4 L/min).
- Dexamethasone (Decadron) 4-8 mg IV q 4 hr may be helpful in HACE, especially when descent is delayed.
- Nifedipine 10 mg tid (Procardia), hydralazine 10-25 mg qid (Apresoline), phentolamine 5-10 mg in 10 mL NS local injection (Regitine), and nitric oxide have been shown to improve HAPE experimentally by lowering pulmonary artery pressure.
- Diuretics, morphine, steroids, and antibiotics have not been shown to improve the symptoms or outcome of HAPE.
- Hyperbaric treatment, if available, is recommended to improve arterial oxygenation and limit the cascade of events that lead to irreparable HACE and/or HAPE.

2.3 Nonfreezing Injuries: Trench Foot (Immersion Foot)

Clin Dermatol 2002;20:445; Arch IM 1991;151:785

Cause: Prolonged exposure of feet to cold in wet footwear.

Epidem: More common in temperatures 32-50°F (0-10°C).

Pathophys:
- No actual freezing of tissue, but injury results from prolonged cooling.
- Three stages of injury:
  1. Ischemic (hours to days)
  2. Hyperemic (days to weeks)
  3. Recovery (weeks to months)

Sx:
- Ischemic phase: cold, tingling followed by numbness, worsening pain, and inability to move foot.
- Hyperemic phase: severe burning pain and reappearance of proximal sensation.
- Recovery phase: hypersensitivity to cold may persist long term; severe cases may lead to permanent disability.

Si:
- Ischemic phase: pale, mottled skin; pulses and sensation are decreased or absent.
- Hyperemic phase: edema, blisters, ulcers; tissue sloughing and gangrene are possible.
- Recovery phase: hyperhidrosis and cold hypersensitivity may persist long term.

Crs:
- Usually complete resolution if treated early.
- Duration of exposure and degree of area involved correlates to length of healing.

Rx:
- Treatment is supportive.
- Gentle warming and drying of affected skin.
- Elevation and soft, clean dry dressings.
- Check for updated tetanus status.
- Wear soft, loose footwear and limit strenuous activities.

2.4   Nonfreezing Injuries: Chilblains (Pernio)

Aviat Space Environ Med 2003;74:564; Clin Sports Med 1989;8:111

Cause: Exposure to cold air or moisture for prolonged period of time.

Epidem:
- More common in women and children.
- Raynaud's disease can predispose to chilblains.

Pathophys: Abnormal peripheral vasoconstrictive response.

Sx:
- Cold, numbness, pain, and pruritis in affected area, usually the extremities or face.

Si:
- Cutaneous manifestations occur up to 12 hr after exposure.
- Initially: localized erythema, cyanosis, nodules, affecting mostly lower extremities, toes, hands, and ears.
- Later: ulceration, vesicles, and bullae.

Crs:
- Usually complete resolution, if treated early.
- Length of exposure correlated to length of healing.
- Affected areas are more prone to reinjury.

Rx:
- Upon rewarming there may be intense pruritis, burning parasthesias, and tender blue nodules, which can persist for 14 d.
- Treatment is mainly supportive.

- Nifedipine (Procardia) 20 mg tid has been shown to have pro-phylactic and therapeutic benefit.
- Topical corticosteroids or a brief oral steroid burst may be beneficial.

2.5 Nonfreezing Injuries: Cold Urticaria

J Am Acad Derm 1992;26:306

Cause: Cold-induced mast cell-mediated generalized urticarial reaction.

Epidem: No age or sex predilection.

Pathophys: IgG-mediated allergic hypersensitivity.

Sx:
- Fatigue, headache, dyspnea, tachycardia.
- Rarely, anaphylactic shock.

Si: Local or generalized wheals, edema, and erythema.

Crs: Recovery is complete, however, individuals may become sensi-tized and be at higher risk at higher temperatures later on.

Lab: Cryoglobulins, cryofibrinogens, cold agglutinins, or hemolysins may be present in a minority of patients.

Other Testing: Ice-water immersion test: immersion of an extremity in an ice bath precipitates angioedema of the distal portion with urticaria at air interface within minutes of the challenge.

Rx:
- Minimize cold exposure: the rate of cooling is more important than the absolute temperature achieved.
- Periactin, doxepin, or hydroxyzine for acute pruritis or urticaria, if severe.
- Fexofenadine (Allegra) 60 mg daily, loratidine (Claritin) 10 mg qd or cetirizine (Zyrtec) 5 mg qd may be beneficial for prophylaxis.

2.6 Freezing Injuries: Frostbite

J Trauma 2004;57:1315; J Trauma 2000;48:171

Cause: Exposure to freezing elements.

Epidem:

- More common in the winter and at higher altitudes.
- Poor acclimitization and failure to anticipate potential for extreme exposures are risk factors affecting outdoor enthusiasts.

Pathophys:

- Intense vasoconstriction occurs as part of the body's temperature-conserving reaction.
- Frostnip is the initial superficial vasoconstrictive response that can lead to frostbite the longer and more extreme the exposure is.
- Frostbite is characterized microscopically as reversible ice crystal formation in the intracellular and extracellular spaces, along with hyperosmolar changes and intracellular damage.
- Three degrees of frostbite are differentiated by the degrees of tissue damage that occur during the rewarming phases:
  First degree: Injury to superficial skin layers.
  Second degree: Injury extends to dermis and subdermis fat cells.
  Third degree: Injury to deeper tissues, including muscle tendon, bone.

Sx:

- Initially, all degrees present similarly with coldness, pain, numbness, and redness.
- Exposed skin is at highest risk, such as the face, ears, fingers.
- Later symptoms may only be anesthesia and paralysis of the affected area.

ENVIRONMENTAL INJURIES

Si:
- Early on, signs indicating the degree of frostbite may not be known until the thawing period has begun.
- Frostnip: digits become hyperemic after thawing, with associated paresthesia, but no evidence of tissue damage or edema.
- First-degree: thawing is painful and associated with erythema and edema. Skin can become waxy in texture at this stage.
- Second-degree: erythema and edema progress into vesicles and straw-colored blisters.
- Third-degree: pain is less severe or nonexistent; blisters may be filled with serosanguineous fluid or frank blood.

Crs:
- Signs of favorable recovery: rapid return to normal temperature, return of sensation, clear blisters, brisk capillary refill time distally, pink skin that blanches.
- Signs of poor recovery: cold, blue tissue without blisters, hard, white insensitive skin; dark red or blue tissue that does not blanch; absence of edema; superimposed trauma; signs of tissue necrosis; and history of freeze-thaw-refreeze.
- Duration of exposure and degree of area involved correlates to length of healing.
- May be hypersensitive to cold weather long term; extra protection against cold exposure and immersion necessary.

Lab: In more severe cases, initial and serial laboratory studies include complete blood count, serum electrolytes, calcium, albumin, amylase, creatine kinase, liver function tests, coagulation studies, and urinalysis.

Other Testing:
- Core temperature monitoring.
- EKG, chest radiograph.
- Patients with severe electrolyte disturbances may require telemetry during initial phase of admission.

Rx:

- Frostnip is best treated with gentle rewarming.
- Other degrees of frostbite require more significant measures:
  - Rapid warming in 45°C (113°F) water bath.
  - Handling and drying of affected skin should be gentle; no massaging of affected areas.
  - Pain medication.
  - Warmed (37°C) intravenous fluids.
  - Avoid ointments, alcohol, tobacco.
  - Elevation of extremities and application of soft, clean dry dressings.
  - Leave blisters alone; broken blisters should be cleaned thoroughly and aloe vera applied.
  - Antibiotics not necessary for minor injury, but penicillin should be considered in a field setting.
  - Tetanus booster should be given.
- Special considerations for advanced-degree frostbite:
  - Referral for sympathectomy, either medical or surgical.
  - Occupational therapy rehabilitation.
  - Amputation in most severe cases.

ENVIRONMENTAL INJURIES

2.7 Hypothermia

Am Fam Phys 2004;70:2325; Med Clin N Amer 1994;78:305; Surg Clin North Amer 1995;75:243; Ann EM 1993;22:370

Cause: Requires two factors: the ambient temperature must be below core body temperature (CBT) and the body's ability to generate heat must be less than ongoing heat losses.

Epidem:
- Hypothermia occurs commonly in water sports (boating, swimming, scuba, white-water rafting), winter sports, and mountaineering.

- It is also quite common in endurance events where the exhausted participant is unable to maintain heat production to overcome environmental losses.
- Major risk factors divided into two categories: those which result in greater heat losses (through impaired thermoregulation) and those leading to reduced thermogenesis. These include age (the very old and young), underlying diseases (cardiovascular, endocrinopathies), exhaustive exercise, alcohol intoxication, and trauma.

Pathophys:
- Heat produced by basal metabolism is adequate to maintain CBT at 37°C (98.6°F) with ambient air temperatures above 28°C (82.4°F). Exercise produces heat allowing thermostasis at lower ambient temperatures.
- Certain environmental conditions can also overwhelm the thermogenic potential, as is seen in cold-water immersion or extreme windchill.
- Heat loss occurs through four transfer processes: conduction, convection, evaporation, and radiation.
- Hypothermia is defined as a core body temperature below 35°C (95°F) and is further divided into: mild (CBT 32-35°C, 89.6-95°F), moderate (CBT 28-32°C, 82.4-89.6°F), and severe (CBT <28°C, 82.4°F).
- Cold affects the function of multiple body systems, including the cardiovascular, pulmonary, urinary, hemocoagulation, and central nervous systems.

Si/Sx:
- Mild hypothermia characterized by tachycardia, uncontrolled shivering, and peripheral vasoconstriction. Cold diuresis, common in the early stages of hypothermia, occurs in response to the increasing central blood pool caused by peripheral vasoconstriction.
- Other findings in mild hypothermia including dysarthria, extremity ataxia, skin pallor, perioral cyanosis, and muscle

rigidity. Deep tendon reflexes are initially brisk, but will diminish as cooling continues.

- With core body temperature below 32°C (89.6°F), the body's ability to respond becomes significantly impaired. The shivering reflex is lost and heat production falls sharply. Hypotension and bradycardia are common, with a 50% reduction in heart rate, at temperatures below 25°C (77°F).
- Worsening cognitive function can contribute further by preventing the victim from recognizing danger and seeking warmth.
- Reduced cerebral blood flow leads to obtundation, stupor, and coma. Pupillary dilation, muscular rigidity, loss of reflexes, and unresponsiveness may lead to the mistaken conclusion that the victim is dead.
- Cardiac arrhythmias become common at CBT below 32°C (89.6°F). Afib frequently occurs in the moderate hypothermic range and is probably due to atrial distention. Supraventricular tachycardia is also common particularly during rewarming. As the temperature falls below 28°C (82.4°F), ventricular irritability leads to more severe arrhythmias including ventricular tachycardia and fibrillation. Spontaneous asystole or fine ventricular fibrillation occurs at temperatures below 20-25°C (68-77°F).

Lab:
- Bleeding time increased.
- BUN increases.
- EKG:
  - EKG changes associated with hypothermia include the arrythmias described above.
  - The Osborne wave ("J" wave) forms at the junction of the QRS complex and T wave giving the ST segment a characteristic "J" shape. It is typically seen at temperatures below 32°C (89.6°F) in leads II and V6 but as temperature falls it becomes prominent in leads V3 and V4. It is reported in

approximately 80% of patients with a CBT below 30°C (86°F).

Crs:

- Aggressive monitoring and fluid replacement are required during rewarming to avoid serious hypovolemic complications.
- One potentially fatal complication during rewarming is CBT afterdrop. Afterdrop refers to the continued core cooling during early rewarming. Two factors contribute to this phenomenon:
    1. Equilibration of blood temperature as the cold blood from the extremities is mobilized and mixes with the central pool (conductive loss).
    2. The cooling of warm blood from the central pool as it perfuses the cold peripheral tissues (convective loss). The temperature drop due to this phenomenon can be significant and may lead to a worsening condition in the face of aggressive rewarming.

Rx:

- Early recognition and prompt rewarming are critical.
- Full recovery, even from extremely low temperature may be possible and full resuscitative efforts should be undertaken even in the severely hypothermic patient.
- Active external rewarming techniques (chemical hot packs, warming blankets or pads, and radiant heat lamps) are usually adequate to warm the mildly hypothermic patient; result in a warming rate of approximately 0.5-1°C/hr, 32.9-33.8°F/hr.
- Internal rewarming refers to the introduction of heat directly to the victim's core.
    - Heated inhalation therapy: use of heated humidified air or oxygen (42-46°C, 108-115°F) delivered through endotracheal tube or mask.
    - IV hydration (isotonic crystalloid solution 5% glucose warmed to 40-42°C, 104-108°F) has dual indication in the

hypothermic patient both as a rewarming technique and to provide intravascular volume replacement.

- Peritoneal lavage: Following the percutaneous placement of an 8 french catheter into the pelvic gutter, warmed isotonic dialysate (40-45°C, 104-113°F) is introduced in allocates of 1-2 L. This fluid is aspirated after 20-30 min. A 6L/hr exchange rate (10-20 cc/kg) results in rewarming at 1-3°/hr.
- Extracorporeal rewarming: This very effective method uses cardiopulmonary bypass equipment for rewarming in the severely hypothermic patients. Advantages with ECR include the ability to control the rate of rewarming and continue tissue perfusion and oxygenation in the setting of cardiac arrest.
- The patient should be handled very gently with continuous cardiac monitoring, as well as close attention to blood pressure. The accurate assessment of the CBT is also crucial. A rectal or esophageal thermistor, placed 15-20 cm into the lumen of the viscera, provides an efficient means for continuous CBT monitoring.
- Arrhythmias: The predominant atrial arrhythmia associated with hypothermia is fibrillation with a slow ventricular response. Afib usually resolves with rewarming and does not require specific therapy. Supraventricular tachyarrhythmias are common during rewarming, but these also resolve as the temperature resolve as the CBT rises. The Ca-channel blockers typically used to treat supraventricular tachyarrhythmias are not effective at low temperatures. Ventricular arrhythmias tend to be resistant to treatment as long as the patient remains cold.
- The decision to stop resuscitative efforts is a complex one. The statement, "A patient isn't dead until they are warm and dead" has shown merit many times in the past with heroic saves of profoundly hypothermic victims.

2.8 Hyperthermia

Crit Care Clin 1999;15:251

Cause: Failure of body's ability to thermoregulate in the face of elevated environmental temperature, extreme physical exertion, and/or disease state affecting the body's ability to effectively dissipate heat.

Epidem:
- More common in the summer and in warm climates.
- Poor acclimatization and failure to anticipate potential for extreme exposures are risk factors affecting outdoor enthusiasts.
- Elderly people, those taking vasoconstrictive drugs, smokers, and extreme athletes are at higher risk.
- Mortality from heatstroke is 10%, usually due to arrhythmia, shock, cardiac ischemia, or renal dysfunction.

Pathophys:
- Inability of the body to effectively thermoregulate causes elevated temperature.
- Evaporative losses worsen dehydration and subsequent sodium loss.
- Electrolyte disturbances lead to muscle breakdown and rhabdomyolysis, which can lead to renal failure.
- The spectrum of heat injury is differentiated by the degrees of systemic changes that develop:
  1. Heat syncope: loss of consciousness characterized by cutaneous vasodilation, with consequent systemic and cerebral hypotension.
  2. Heat cramps: muscular cramps caused by electrolyte and fluid depletion.
  3. Heat exhaustion: fatigue, weakness, and other systemic symptoms resulting from prolonged heat exposure, dehydration, and electrolyte depletion.

4. Heatstroke: life-threatening cerebral dysfunction resulting from a failure of the thermoregulatory mechanism.

Sx:

- Symptoms of heat injuries are common to all categories and grow worse as duration of exposure and delay of treatment increase:
  1. Heat syncope: fatigue, thirst, lightheadedness, and headache.
  2. Heat cramps: muscular cramps, pain, and spasms.
  3. Heat exhaustion: fatigue, weakness, anxiety, impaired judgment, hyperventilation, and other systemic symptoms.
  4. Heatstroke: impaired consciousness, nausea, and seizures.

Si:

- Absence of sweating reflects advanced injury and the highest risk for heatstroke.
- Symptoms of heat injuries progress from mild discomfort to systemic compromise with increasing temperature:
  1. Heat syncope: rapid pulse and hypotension.
  2. Heat cramps: skin moist and cool, profuse sweating, palpable muscle twitching, normal to slightly elevated core temperature.
  3. Heat exhaustion: core temperature $>37.8°C$ (100°F), rapid pulse, mental status changes.
  4. Heatstroke: high fever ($>41°C$, 106°F), seizure activity, delirium, rhabdomyolysis.

Crs:

- Signs of favorable recovery: rapid return to normal temperature, maintenance of isotonic volume, lack of central nervous systemic symptoms.
- Signs of poor recovery: delayed removal from hot environment, prolonged dehydration, electrolyte disturbance, coexisting morbidity (age, heart disease, obesity, trauma).

- Exertional heat injury, such as that experienced by marathon runners and triathletes, carries a more favorable prognosis.
- Previous heat injury is a risk for subsequent injury and should be considered in risk prevention.

Lab:
- Initial tests: urinalysis to demonstrate ketonuria and early dehydration, renal function tests, and serum sodium.
- Later tests: serial urinalysis, urine myoglobin, serum chemistries to include potassium, phosphorus, and calcium, creatine kinase, complete blood count.
- Consider blood alcohol level and screening for illicit substances.

Other Testing:
- Core temperature monitoring.
- EKG: ST changes suggesting ischemia, peaked T waves of hyperkalemia.
- Patients with severe electrolyte disturbances may require telemetry during initial hospitalization.

Rx:
- Heat syncope is treated with rest, sitting in a cool place, and oral fluid rehydration.
- Heat cramps are treated as above, but intravenous fluids may be necessary to deliver sufficient isotonic saline more rapidly.
- Sodium tablets are not recommended because of their slow absorption.
- Heat exhaustion is treated as above, but also includes more aggressive initial intravenous fluid replacement (1-2 L over 2-4 hr) and more prolonged therapy (up to 24 hr).
- Intravenous 3% (hypertonic) saline may be necessary if sodium depletion is severe.
- There are three major considerations for treating heatstroke:

1. Initially: rapid cooling to bring the core temperature to below 39°C (102°F), using ice baths, fans, and cold compresses.
   - Gastric lavage and submersion are minimally effective, but not recommended because of practicality and interference with monitoring.
   - Antipyretics are not effective for environmentally-induced hyperthermia and are contraindicated.
   - Antiseizure medication is probably not necessary until the core temperature is reduced (chlorpromazine 25-50 mg or diazepam 5-10 mg intravenously can be helpful in this regard).
2. Management of shock—both hypovolemic and/or cardiogenic, is critical.
   - Central venous pressure monitoring may be necessary to allow rapid, aggressive volume replacement without overloading the circulation.
3. Close monitoring for systemic complications, such as rhabdomyolysis, renal failure, DIC, cardiac arrhythmias, and serious electrolyte disturbances is key.
   - Fluid administration should be sufficient to maintain high urine output (>50 mL/hr).
   - Use of mannitol (0.25 mg/kg) and alkalinizing the urine (intravenous sodium bicarbonate, 250 mL of 4%) should be considered.

Chapter 3

Nutrition and Ergogenics

3.1 General

Nutrition guidelines are established every 5 years by the U.S. Department of Agriculture and the U.S. Department of Health and Human Services (http://www.nalusda.gov/fnic/dga/dguide95.html). The Food Guide Pyramid (http://www.nal.usda.gov:8001/py/pmap. htm) offers a general guide for a healthy diet (see Table 3.1).

Table 3.1 Nutrition Guide for Optimum Performance

Eat a high carbohydrate diet.
Taper by decreasing the intensity and/or duration of practice for 1-2 d before
  competition.
Eat a carbohydrate meal 3-4 hr before competition.
Maintain adequate fluid intake before and during competition.
Avoid sugar less than 1 hr before competition.
After exhausting exercise, eat carbohydrates.
Eat foods containing adequate vitamins and minerals.

Banned Drugs

- For the most current list of drugs banned by the National Collegiate Athletic Association (NCAA) and the International Olympic Committee, check the websites:
  - http://www.ncaa.org/sports_sciences/drugtesting/ banned_list.html
  - http://www.olympic.org/ioc/e/org/medcom/medcom_ antidopage_e.html

3.2 Creatine

Prim Care 2005;32:277; Ped Clin North Am 2002;49:435, 2002; 49:829; Clin Sports Med 1999;18:651; Nut Aspects of Ex 1999;18:651; Phy Sportsmed 1999;27:47

Pathophys:

- Short-burst, intense exercise rapidly consumes ATP.
- Phosphocreatine serves as an energy buffer, transferring its phosphate group to ADP to regenerate ATP.
- There is 4-6× more creatine phosphate (CP) than ATP stored in cells.
- Both of these energy sources are depleted within 6-10 secs of intensive exercise, and they are replenished primarily through breakdown of carbohydrates and fats.
- Ergogenic effects:
  - Creatine stores in muscle are increased through the ingestion of creatine (at most about 20%).
  - Increasing the supply of creatine phosphate provides more energy to exercising muscle.
  - Creatine improves performance in short-duration, repetitive, and intense exercise. Improvement in cycling, swimming, kayaking, rowing, weight lifting, jumping and sprinting ability have been shown.
  - Creatine increases total body mass and fat-free muscle mass (0.5-2.0 kg).
  - Creatine decreases lactic acid levels in the blood during sprints.
  - Conversely, creatine does not improve isometric strength, power, or aerobic endurance.
  - Middle-aged athletes may benefit more than younger athletes.
  - Men seem to benefit more than women from creatine use.
  - Simultaneous training exercise is required for a beneficial effect.

- Creatine use with exercise results in increases in muscle mass. Type I (slow twitch, aerobic), type IIA (intermediate, anaerobic), and type IIB (fast twitch, anaerobic) muscle mass are increased.
- Caffeine reduces the efficacy of creatine.
- Large carbohydrate intake augments muscle uptake of creatine.
- Best effects seen in subjects with lower initial creatine stores (vegetarians)

Sx: Muscle cramps (25% of users), strains, decrease urine output, diarrhea.

Cmplc: There are some reports of association with exertional rhab-domyolysis (J Am Board Fam Pract 2000;13:134) and heat injuries probably related to poor hydration, cardiac arrhythmia, cardiomyopathy, DVT, seizure, and use of other ergogenic substances.

Lab: UA, BUN/Cr or other labs indicated by presentation.

Rx:
- A loading dose of 0.3 gm/kg of body weight per day (0.14 gm/lb of body weight per day) divided over 4-5 doses/d is taken for 5-7 d.
- A maintenance dose of 0.03 gm/kg of body weight per day (0.014 gm/lb of body weight per day) is subsequently taken.
- Naturally available creatine is found in beef, dairy products, and fish.
- Not recommended for adolescents.

3.3　Anabolic Steroids

Prim Care 2005;32:277; Ped Clin North Am 2002;49:829; Clin Sports Med 1999;18:667; Am J Sports Med 1993;21:468; Clin Sports Med 1998;17:299

Cause: Oral or injectable supplementation.

Epidem: 6.6% of HS male seniors; mean age to start 14; also used by the recreational athlete looking for rapid gains.

Pathophys:
- Testosterone is produced in the testes and adrenals.
- Androstenedione is produced in the adrenal gland and testes then converted in the liver to testosterone.
- Testosterone affects almost all body tissues by decreasing tissue breakdown and increasing tissue production.
- Excess testosterone is peripherally converted to estrogen, resulting in feminization in males (Ann Pharm 1992;26:520).
- Size and strength gains through anticatabolic, anabolic, and motivational effects.
  - Anticatabolic: displacement of cortisol from receptors resulting in less wasting and negative nitrogen balance.
  - Anabolic effect: induce protein synthesis; stimulation of endogenous HGH.
  - Motivational: aggressiveness to train hard.
- Effects are reversed as soon as the steroids are stopped.

Sx: Significant improvement in performance more than indicated by level of training; muscle hypertrophy; aggressiveness and mood swings to include paranoia, mania, and hypomania; risk-taking behaviors; premature cardiovascular disease.

Si: Muscular hypertrophy; acne; striae; elevated BP; gynecomastia; gonadal atrophy, and impaired spermatogenesis; clitorimegaly; male pattern baldness.

Cmplc: Sudden death, myocardial infarction, increased low-density lipoproteins (LDLs), decreased high-density lipoproteins (HDLs), hypertension, concentric cardiac hypertrophy, hypercoagulability, decreased spermatogenesis, decreased testicle size, prostate hypertrophy, prostate cancer, voice alterations, liver damage and cancer, premature epiphyseal closure with resulting short stature, weaker tendons (Achilles and patellar tendon rupture), electrolyte imbalances, insulin resistance, skin pathology, aggression, depression, paranoia, HIV, and hep B and C.

Lab: Sperm count, electrolytes, glucose, serum lipids, coagulation studies, liver function tests, PSA (over 40 or 50 years of age), an electrocardiogram, and possibly an echocardiogram if indications of ventricular hypertrophy are present; screening for hep B, hep C, and HIV is recommended for any athlete using injectable drugs. Urine screen is done to measure testosterone:epitestosterone ratio; >6 is a positive test.

Rx:
- Stop supplementation.
- Management of poststeroid depressive sx and dependence sx.
- Multidisciplinary management approach.

3.4 Human Growth Hormone

Prim Care 2005;32:277; J Clin Endo and Met 1999;84:3591; Am J Sports Med 1993;21:468

Cause: Supplementation by injection.

Epidem: Unknown.

Pathophys:
- Growth hormone (somatotropin) is produced in the anterior pituitary gland.
- The level of growth hormone increases with exercise and hypoglycemia.
- This increase may not occur in obese athletes (J Clin Endo and Met 1999;84:3156).
- Growth hormone increases liver and osteoblast production of insulin-like growth factor (ILGF-I) that has anabolic properties.
- Ergogenic effects:
  - Growth hormone inhibits glucose breakdown and increases the level of free fatty acids that can be used for energy.

NUTRITION AND
ERGOGENICS

- Growth hormone increases muscle mass, strength, and endurance.
- Growth hormone decreases body fat.
- Growth hormone may also increase cardiac output and sweating to help in cooling.

Sx: Signs of acromegaly (increased skull size with prominent cheekbones, protruding jaw and frontal bossing, spade-like hands), arthralgias, impotence.

Si: Signs of CHF, lung sounds for pulmonary edema, joints for arthritis, lymph glands, face and extremities for swelling, hair loss, weight, eye examination for papilledema, prostate mass (digital rectal examination), insulin resistance.

Lab:
- Prostate-specific antigen (over 40 or 50 years of age), bone age for premature closure of epiphyses, glucose, and serum lipids; monitoring for hep B, hep C, and HIV is indicated in athletes using needles for administration.
- Current assays to detect abuse of recombinant human growth hormone are of insufficient sensitivity and specificity to prove useful, especially in light of the large fluctuations that may be greater than 100-fold in athletes.
- Collagen and procollagen markers are being studied as possible tests for abuse.

Cmplc:
- Acromegaly, prostate cancer (Science 1998;279:563), hypertension, heart failure, and arthritis.
- Though not well studied, short-term use of growth hormone may result in sodium and fluid retention, flushing, or a feeling of heaviness in the legs.
- Osteoporosis, impotence/amenorrhea, myopathy, hypertension, diabetes, peripheral neuropathy.
- HIV, hep B and C.
- Significant cost (up to $30,000/yr).

Rx: Stop supplementation and screen for complications.

3.5 Erythropoietin (EPO and rEPO)

Prim Care 2005;32:277; Neurol 2002;58:665; Am J Sports Med
     1996;24:PS004

Cause: iv or SQ supplementation.

Epidem: Increased use with availability of rEPO.

Pathophys:

- EPO is manufactured through an enzyme produced in adult
  kidneys and fetal livers.
- Erythropoietin is produced in response to hypoxia, and it stim-
  ulates bone marrow production of erythrocytes.
- A synthetic recombinant erythropoietin (rEPO) is available
- Ergogenic effects:
  - Erythropoietin use results in higher hematocrit, muscle
    glycogen, and free fatty acids.
  - After endurance exercise, lactic acid levels are lower.
  - Erythropoietin used in athletes for 6 wk was shown to
    increase maximal oxygen consumption (VO_{2max}) and
    endurance.
  - Before the advent of rEPO, transfusion with 1-2 L of blood
    also resulted in increased maximal oxygen uptake and
    performance.

Sx: Headache, sx of DVT/PE, exertional collapse.

Si: Hypertension, signs of DVT/PE.

Cmplc: Myalgia, hyperviscosity, hypercoagulability, hypertension, and
     dehydration; DVT, PE, CVA, sudden death.

Lab: Suggested monitoring should include hemoglobin and hematocrit
     at minimum; other laboratory studies for hep B, hep C, and HIV
     should be included for athletes using intravenous medications.

NUTRITION AND
ERGOGENICS

Diff Dx: Blood doping or altitude training effect; polycythemia vera.

Rx: Stop the supplementation and monitor for complications.

3.6 Stimulants

Ped Clin N Amer 2002;49:433; 2002;49:829; Clin Sports Med 1997;16:375; The Hughston Clinic Sports Medicine Book. Baltimore: Williams & Wilkins, 1995.

Cause: Oral supplementation or ingestion of caffeine, amphetamines, ephedra.

Epidem: Widespread use in all sports (esp caffeine).

Pathophys:
- Caffeine is a xanthine derivative.
- Ephedra is found naturally in plants like *ma huang* and *Sida cordifolia*, found in purified forms as ephedrine, pseudoephedrine, PPA, and sold as "Ripped Fuel," "Hydroxycut," "Metabolife." If manufactured in herbal or extract form, can be sold as a dietary supplement without FDA regulations.
- Stimulants enhance mental alertness and possess sympathomimetic effects.
- Increases release of FFA from adipose cells.
- Enhances contractility of skeletal and cardiac muscle.
- Ergogenic effects:
  - More recent studies of amphetamines show no increased performance in sprint and middle distance running, sprint and middle distance swimming, combination cycling and running endurance, endurance while bench stepping with weights, or reaction time.
  - Studies of stimulants have shown no performance enhancing effects at recommended doses (Clin J Sp Med 1997;7:168) but may have some benefit at higher doses or when combined with caffeine (Br J Clin Pharm 2000;50:205; Eur J Appl Phys 1998;77:427).

- In 1983, the FDA banned all over-the-counter (OTC) drugs that included both synthetic ephedrine and caffeine, due to serious adverse side effects. They are still commonly used together as dietary supplements that combine natural ephedra with guarana or kola nut, both natural forms of caffeine.
- Ephedra has been shown to have no weight-loss effects on nonobese people.
- Caffeine, on the other hand, improved endurance cycling performance by 19.5%.
- Fat use is increased, and carbohydrate use decreased.
- Nicotine in smokeless tobacco may decrease strength and power.

Sx:

- Aerobic exercise intolerance (rapid rise in HR).
- Palpitations, psychosis, restlessness, dizziness, insomnia, motor tics, dry mouth, diarrhea or constipation, anorexia, impotence, or change in libido.
- Cocaine causes excitement, restlessness, anxiety, confusion, increased sympathetic tone, nausea, vomiting, abdominal pain, seizures, elevated body temperature, chills, and unconsciousness.
- Caffeine may cause headache, excitement, agitation, tinnitus, tremors, palpitations, and even seizures.
- Sympathomimetics may cause anxiety, agitation, paranoia, hypertension, and palpitations.
- PPA taken off shelves due to increased risk of hemorrhagic stroke in women.

Si: Hypertension, tachycardia, arrhythmia, mental confusion, tremor.

Cmplc: Arrhythmia with complication, MI, seizure, CVA/TIA, sudden death, weight loss.

Lab:

- Urine vanillylmandelic acid (VMA), metanephrines, and 5-hydroxyindoleacetic acid (5-HIAA) levels may be increased

with caffeine use, leading to a misdiagnosis of pheochromocytoma; EKG to eval rythm.
- Caffeine is legal, but there are limits to the amounts; IOC and
NCAA have urinary threshold of <12 mcg/ml and 15 mcg/ml,
respectively.

Diff Dx: Pheochromocytoma, anxiety state.

Rx:

- Caffeine is probably ergogenic between 250-350 mg, which is
found in approximately 1-2 cups of regular coffee or 5-7 cans of
caffeinated soda taken 1 hr before exercise.
  - The maximum safe dosage of caffeine even for emergency
  indications is approximately 500 mg per dose or 2500 mg/d.
- Stop/withhold other stimulants when more symptomatic.

3.7 HMB (Beta-Hydroxy-Beta-Methylbutyrate)

Prim Care 2005;32:277; J Appl Phys 2003;94:651; J Appl Phys
2000;89:1340; Phy Sportsmed 1997;25:76; Nutrition 2000;16:734

Cause: Oral supplementation.

Epidem: Body builders, distance runners.

Pathophys:

- Metabolite of the essential amino acid leucine.
- Endogenously made, but also found in catfish, breastmilk, and
citrus fruits.
- Decrease nitrogen and protein loss by inhibiting protein
breakdown.
- Ergogenic effects:
  - Hypothesized that high level of HMB decreases protein
  catabolism thus creating an anabolic effect.

- HMB contributes to increasing strength and lean muscle mass in resistance training as well as lessening the amount of muscle damage during endurance activities.
- Both animal and a number of double-blinded, placebo controlled human studies have shown evidence to support these theories.
- Preliminary studies have shown only modest improvement in body strength and fat-free muscle mass in untrained individuals taking HMB compared to placebo.
- Nissen et al found a significant decrease in urinary muscle breakdown products and a significant increase in fat-free muscle mass and strength in those taking 1.5-3.0 gm/day compared to placebo during a 4-wk intense resistance training program (J Appl Physiol 1996;81:2095).
- Knitter et al also found a significant decrease in serum levels of CPK and LDH, both indicators of muscle damage, after a 20-km run in those taking 3 gm/day compared to placebo for 6 wk prior to the run (J Appl Physiol 2000;89:1340).

Sx: Well-tolerated without known side effects in short-term studies; studies have shown to actually decrease cholesterol values and lower systolic blood pressure.

Complc: Long-term effects unknown; study results still preliminary.

Rx: One gm, tid.

3.8 Chromium Picolinate

Phy Sportsmed 1997;25:76; Am J Sports Med 2002;30:907

Cause: Oral supplementation.

Pathophys:
- Essential trace mineral present in foods such as mushrooms, prunes, nuts, whole grains, and cereals,
- Has a low absorption from gi tract, so it is combined and sold as chromium picolinate to aid absorption.

- Enhances the activity of insulin and thought to improve glucose tolerance, lipid profiles, and amino acid incorporation into muscles.
- Ergogenic effects:
  - Promoted to decrease body fat and increase lean muscle mass.
  - Became popular after knowledge that chromium excretion was believed to increase during exercise, putting athletes at risk for chromium deficiency, clinical fatigue, and weight gain.
  - This decrease is also associated with metabolic disturbances of increased insulin levels and decreased glucose tolerance.
  - Early studies showed athletes to decrease their body fat and increase muscle mass from supplementation of 200 mcg/d (Int J Sp Nutr 1992;2:343; Int J Biosoc Med Res 1989; 11:163).
  - Measurement techniques in these studies, however, have come into question, and more recent studies have failed to demonstrate any significant benefits (Med Sci Sports Exerc 1996;28:139).

Si: N/A.

Sx: At doses between 50-200 mcg/d taken less than 1 month, only GI side effects have been reported.

Complc:
- Anemia, cognitive impairment, chromosome damage, and interstitial nephritis have been reported with increased dosages and/or duration.
- Given the lack of convincing evidence and known long-term side effects, the use of chromium as an ergogenic aid should not be recommended.

Rx: No RDA recommendation; 50-200 mcg/d.

3.9   Branched Chain Amino Acids (BCAA)

J Nutr 2004;134:1583S; Amer J Clin Nutrition 2000;72; Amer J
    Sports Med 2002;30:907

Cause: Oral ingestion of essential amino acids leucine, isoleucine, and
    valine. Recommended daily intake is 3 gm/d; available in tablet
    or powder form.

Epidem: Endurance athletes.

Pathophys:
- Exercise induces oxidation of BCAA in skeletal muscle.
- BCAA are energy substrates for the citric acid cycle and for
  gluconeogenesis.
- Leucine is found to promote muscle protein synthesis when
  administered to animals.
- Ergogenic effects:
  - Supplementation before and after exercise to decrease
    exercise-induced muscle damage and promote muscle
    synthesis.
  - Increase mental endurance and decrease performance fatigue
    by being a factor in the central fatigue hypothesis (see 21.1).
    This suggests that increased levels of serotonin in the brain
    can lead to fatigue during prolonged exercise. BCAA being
    taken from the blood and oxidized in skeletal muscle during
    exercise frees more tryptophan to cross the BBB, leading to
    higher serotonin levels and increased fatigue. It is theorized
    that increasing BCAA levels in the blood will compete with
    tryptophan transport mechanisms.
    N.B. Science behind this hypothesis is still unclear.
    Ergogenic effects of high levels of BCAA have not been
        proven.

Sx: GI upset most common; can also inhibit absorption of other
    amino acids and cause gastric water retention; long-term effects
    not determined.

NUTRITION AND ERGOGENICS

Cmplc: Competition with amino acids for transport into the brain and may lower neurotransmitter synthesis, although significance of this is unknown; no evidence of carcinogenesis or that BCAA supplementation results in such high levels to reproduce neurologic damage seen with MSUD.

Rx: Available in powder/tablet; usually combined with other amino acids; recommended supplement at 5-10 gm/d prior to exercise.

3.10 Dehydroepiandrosterone (DHEA)/Androstenedione (Andro)

Clin Sports Med 2004;23:255; Ped Clin North Am 2002;49:435

Cause: Oral ingestion of supplement.

Epidem: Body builder, strength training.

Pathophys:

- Natural androgen produced by the adrenal glands and testes. It is a precursor to testosterone and estrogen.
- Thought to increase levels of testosterone, IGF-1 (insulin-like growth factor 1), and human growth hormone.
- Promoted to enhance physical power, increase muscle mass.
- Enhance physiologic well-being in men >50 y/o.
- Most studies have been focused on men >50 y/o to market DHEA as an OTC antiaging supplement. Studies on younger athletes (<30 y/o) are limited and have failed to prove any physical or performance benefit.
- Has not been proven to increase testosterone levels.
- Andro (androstenedione): Another prohormone in the testosterone/estrogen pathway with claims to increase strength and improve performance. Like DHEA, andro shows a similar side effect profile and studies have been unable to prove benefits. Attention was given to andro in the 1960s when initial studies showed increases in serum testosterone in females, but more

recent studies have failed to duplicate this result and many
have even shown increases in serum estrogen levels. It is also a
banned substance.

Sx: Similar to anabolic steroids: gynecomastia, hirsutism/alopecia,
acne, increased LDL; has the potential to increase risk for
prostate and endometrial cancer.

Lab: Detected through increased testosterone:epitestosterone ratio
(6:1), which gives a positive screen for steroids (see 3.3).

3.11 Glutamine

Ped Clin North Am 2002;49:435; Clin Sports Med 1999;18:633; Clin
J Sport Med 1999;18:667

Cause: Nonessential amino acid; most abundant amino acid in human
muscle; also found in peanuts, soybeans, almonds.

Epidem: Unknown.

Pathophys:
- Important factor in the optimal function of certain cells of the
immune system.
- Has been shown to increase release of HGH and ACTH but
has not been studied much as an ergogenic advantage in this
regard.
- Ergogenic effects:
  - Research has shown that prolonged, intensive exercise
decreases glutamine and this could impair an athlete's
immunologic response.
  - Theorized that plasma glutamine could be an indicator for
an athlete being overtrained or being immune impaired and
that supplementation could help prevent this injury (see
21.1).

- Both animal and human studies ha
  ve not shown consistent benefits to supplemental glutamine.

Sx: Few when taken in small/RDA recommended amounts; gi side effects most common, but metabolic disturbances and reactions to impurities found in various supplements have been reported.

Rx: 2 gm/d.

Chapter 4

Cervical Spine Injuries

4.1 Cervical Strain/Sprain

Ligamentous Sprain, Neck Strain, Whiplash, Myofascial Neck Pain

Prim Care 2004;31:19; Phy Sportsmed 1997;25:60; Current Diagnosis and Treatment in Family Medicine. McGraw-Hill, New York 2004:297

Cause: Strain is injury to muscle-tendon unit. Sprain is ligamentous or capsular injury.

Epidem: Often due to rapid and excessive range of motion in one or more planes; falls, motor vehicle accidents.

Pathophys:
- The anterior longitudinal ligament prevents hyperextension. Injury to this ligament results in a "whiplash."
- The posterior longitudinal ligament prevents hyperflexion.
- Additional support is provided by the ligamentum flavum, interspinous ligaments, ligamentum nuchae.
- Soft-tissue injury involving these supportive muscles and ligaments of the neck.
- Normal ROM:
  - Flexion 60°, extension 70°, lateral flexion 45°, rotation 80°.

Sx:
- Nonradicular neck and shoulder pain worsened by motion of neck.
- Decreased cervical range of motion.

Si: Decreased range of motion in multiple directions. Spasm of local musculature may be present. No neurologic dysfunction or bony tenderness.

Crs: Self-limited. Most symptoms resolve completely within 4-6 wk.

Cmplc: Chronic pain and disability; cervical spine instability; HNP; spondylosis or acquired cervical spinal stenosis with or without myelopathy.

Diff Dx: Cervical spondylosis (see 4.2); cervical fracture; cervical radiculopathy (see 4.3); meningitis; myofascial pain.

X-ray: Basic assessment with a 3-view series (AP, lateral, odontoid); consider lateral flexion/extension views to r/o instability for severe, persistent pain or a severe mechanism (abn include >3.5-mm horizontal displacement with adjacent vertebrae or 11° rotational difference).

Rx:
- Rest, anti-inflammatory medications.
- Ice massage.
- Consider short-term rest neck in a soft collar.
- Muscle relaxants may be indicated.
- Range-of-motion rehabilitation when tolerated and a strengthening program starting with isometrics then isotonic exercises.
- Focus on posture during activity and esp at work and while driving.

Return to Activity: Only when asymptomatic, normal muscle strength, and pain-free full cervical range of motion is present. There should be no neck pain with and without axial compression or Spurling's.

4.2 Cervical Spondylosis / Spinal Stenosis

Cervical Spine Degenerative Disc Disease, Cervical Spine Degenerative Joint Disease, Osteoarthritis

Ortho Clin North Am 2002;33:329; Am Fam Phys 2000;62:1064; Clin Sports Med 1990;9:279; Clin Sports Med 1998;17:121

Cause: Ingrowth of bony spurs or herniation of disc material.

Epidem: Cervical spine stenosis increases the risk of permanent neurologic injury. Highest risk of injury in athletes participating in contact and collision sports.

Pathophys:
- Spondylosis is degeneration of intervertebral discs and facet joints with subsequent osteophytic encroachment.
- Cervical spinal stenosis is developmental narrowing of the AP diameter of the cervical canal or secondary to spondylosis and degenerative disease.
- Narrowing (stenosis) of the spinal canal or neural foramen with restriction/ compression of the spinal cord or nerve roots.
- Loss of normal cerebral spinal fluid cushion around the cord or deformation of the cord.
- These changes can result in nerve root symptoms or cord encroachment.
- Cord changes from pressure result in myelopathy, with upper motor neuron symptoms in the lower extremity.

Sx:
- Chronic neck pain, stiffness, and crepitus with normal motion.
- Reduce cervical ROM.
- Radicular upper extremity symptoms.
- Myelopathy with upper motor neuron symptoms of spasticity, gait disturbance, hyperreflexia or in advanced cases, bladder symptoms.

Si:
- Tenderness to palpation along lateral neck or along the spinous processes.
- Limitations of neck motion.
- Positive Spurling's (see 4.3).
- Evaluate the motor and sensory function of the upper extremity and DTRs in the LE (see 4.3).

Crs: Usually a progressive process, although it is difficult to predict who will progress.

Cmplc:
- May develop quadriparesis due to central cord syndrome (contusion of central portion of spinal cord).
- Transient quadriplegia/cervical cord neuropraxia is an acute transient neurologic episode of cervical cord origin. Findings include both arms, legs, all four extremities, or an ipsilateral arm and leg. Sensory changes are present with or without motor findings.
- Probability or recurrence depends on spinal canal/vertebral body ratio.

Diff Dx: Burner/stinger (see 4.5), herniated cervical disc (see 4.4), cervical fracture.

Lab: If radicular symptoms present, may consider EMG.

X-ray:
- Radiographs may see sclerosis in the intervertebral disc area with osteophytes. Osteophytes may project from the posterior portion of the vertebral body into the spinal canal, causing stenosis. Should evaluate Torg (or Pavlov's) ratio of spinal canal diameter to vertebral body diameter. Ratio <0.8 implies spinal stenosis.
- MRI evaluation of spinal cord diameter to canal diameter is more reliable; also evaluate for cervical cord signal indicating cord compromise and myelomalacia.

Rx:
- Rest, nonsteroidal anti-inflammatory medications and observation if symptoms resolving.
- Steroids may be indicated (short course: ie, prednisone 60 mg/d for 5-7 days) for acute pain exacerbations.
- Occasional consultation to a pain clinic for epidural steroid injections.
- Neurosurgical consult if any complications, recurrent symptoms, or cervical cord problems/findings.

Return to Activity: Depends on symptomatology and results of radiographic evaluation. Generally pain-free ROM and normal strength. Patients with cervical stenosis should avoid high-impact activities and those requiring and involving repetitive flexion and extension.

4.3   Cervical Radiculopathy

Clin Sports Med 2002;21:37; Phy Sportsmed 1997;25:60

Cause: Disc protrusion, which may result in nerve root or spinal cord impingement.

Epidem: Acute injury from compression or hyperflexion injury. Chronic symptoms due to degeneration of disc.

Pathophys:
- C2 through C7 are connected in series with intervertebral discs between each vertebral body.
- Intervertebral discs are composed of an annulus fibrosis (strong fibrous ring) that surrounds the nucleus pulposus.
- Nerve roots exit one each side between the bodies and the transverse processes of adjoining vertebrae (each nerve root exits above the cervical level, ie, C5 exits between C4 and C5).
- Acute injury due to rupture of the disc where nucleus pulposus extrudes through a tear in the annulus fibrosus.

- Chronic symptoms from degeneration of the disc with combination of disc and osteophytic encroachment on the nerve foramen.

Sx: Neck pain with radiation into shoulder or arm. Burning pain, weakness, or sensory changes in the distribution of a specific nerve root. May have upper motor neuron sx in the LE, ie, bowel or bladder sx).

Si: Reproduction of symptoms with compression test or Spurling's maneuver. Pain relieved with distraction test. May isolate weakness or neurologic deficits (reflex and/or sensory).
- Compression test:
  - Examiner applies axial load by applying pressure to the patient's head.
  - Positive test indicated by reproduction of radicular sx.
- Spurling's test (Figure 4.1):
  - Examiner gently extends and laterally flexes the neck.
  - Positive test indicated by ipsiateral radicular sx.
- Distraction test:
  - Examiner provides axial traction of the c-spine to relieve radicular sx.
- Motor function tests (see Table 4.1):

Table 4.1   Motor Function Tests

Nerve Root	Muscle	Functional Test
C1-2		flexion of the head
C3		lateral bending of the head
C4	trapezius	shoulder shrug
C5	deltoid	shoulder abduction
C5-6	biceps	elbow flexion
C6	extensor carpi radialis	wrist extension
C7	triceps, finger extensors	elbow extension, finger extension
C8	flexor digitorum	finger flexion
C8-T1	interosseous muscles	finger abduction

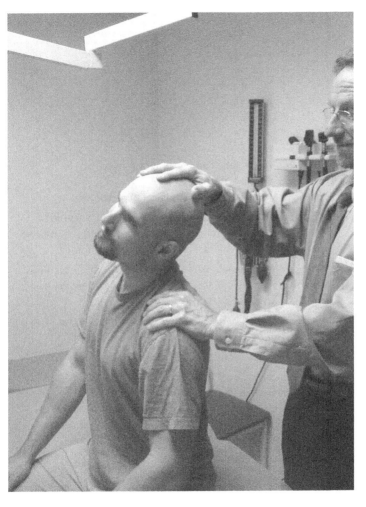

Figure 4.1 Spurling's Test

- Dermatome distribution tests:
  - C2   upper neck/occiput
  - C3   lower neck
  - C4   shoulder tip
  - C5   lateral arm (deltoid area)
  - C6   lateral forearm and thumb
  - C7   middle finger
  - C8   medial forearm and little finger
- Reflex testing:
  - C5-C6   biceps reflex and brachioradialis reflex
  - C7-C8   triceps reflex

Evaluate gait and LE DTRs for signs of hyperreflexia.

Crs: Symptoms usually respond to conservative therapy within 6-12 wks. If severe neurologic deficits or symptoms persist despite conservative management, surgical consult is warranted.

Cmplc: Progressive encroachment upon nerve root with escalating symptomatology. Association with chronic, recurrent cervical nerve root neuropraxia (burner).

Diff Dx: Cervical spinal stenosis (see 4.2), demyelinating conditions, Singer or Burner (see 4.4), thoracic outlet syndrome.

Lab: EMG and NCS to determine nerve root involved and extent.

X-ray:

- Radiographs may show disc space narrowing, anterior bony ridging, and loss of normal cervical lordosis.
- CT not very useful in visualizing cervical disc pathology.
- MRI to display compression.

Rx:

- Rest, NSAIDs, muscle relaxants, and/or pain control.
- If radicular symptoms present, short course of oral steroids may be indicated (prednisone 60 mg/d for 5-7 days).
- Cervical traction either through physical therapy or home traction devices may offer relief.

- Gentle active ROM, avoid extremes of flexion and extension.
- Spinal manipulation should be avoided.

Return to Activity: Normal or near normal nonpainful ROM, normal neurologic exam, and negative Spurling's.

4.4 Transient Brachial Plexopathy (Burner, Stinger)

Clin Sports Med 2003;22:49; Am Fam Phys 1999;60:2035; Phy Sportsmed 1997;25:60; 1996;24:57

Cause: Neurologic insult to the brachial plexus or cervical nerve root.

Epidem: The most common neurologic cervical injury. Traction injury to shoulder or compression injury to the neck. Common in contact sports such as football and wrestling. Most commonly involves C5-C6 nerve distribution.

Pathophys: A transient, unilateral neuropraxia due to traction of the brachial plexus or compression of the cervical nerve root. More severe lesions may be due to axonotmesis or neurotmesis.

Sx: Intense sharp, unilateral "burning" paresthesia or weakness in the upper extremity.

Si: Neurologic dysfunction in sensory and motor may be present but usually resolves within minutes (most motor findings are in a C5 or C6 distribution). Spurling's maneuver (see 4.4) positive in compression and negative in traction injury.

Crs:
- Initially patients are overtly symptomatic; yet show quick recovery of paresthesia and/or weakness with full range of motion without pain.
- Recurrent stingers in close proximity will result in more profound symptoms lasting longer because of incomplete recovery of the brachial plexus.

Cmplc: Cervical cord neuropraxia; nonreversible nerve injury.

Diff Dx: Herniated disc (see 4.4); cervical stenosis (see 4.3).

Lab: EMG warranted for persistent symptoms.

X-ray: MRI of the cervical spine if persistent neurologic deficit and prolonged or recurrent symptoms.

Rx:
- Remove from activity until all symptoms resolve.
- If injury occurred from axial load injury or bilateral should warrant urgent evaluation.
- Recurrent symptoms (>3 episodes) or sx lasting > 24 hr should be evaluated with imaging studies (MRI) to rule out cervical spine stenosis or HNP.
- Prevention includes strengthening program for neck and protective neck collar.
- While symptomatic, athletes should avoid further injury to the brachial plexus:
  - No back-pack wear, weight lifting, or any traction on the affected arm.
  - Avoid repetitive flexion-extension activities.

Return to Activity: Pain-free cervical ROM, normal strength (focus on C5, C6), and negative Spurling's. Recurrent acute and chronic burners are a relative contraindication to contact sports (Clin J Sport Med 1997;7:273).

4.5   Cervical Instability

Clin Sports Med 2003;22:513; 1998;17:137

Cause: Injury and disruption of the ligaments supporting the vertebral bodies.

Epidem: Potentially catastrophic injury. Often due to rapid and excessive/forceful range of cervical motion in one or more planes.

Pathophys: Injury to the supportive ligaments of the cervical spine with potential for progressive instability, cervical spine deformity, and spinal cord injury. May result in dislocation with compromise of cervical cord. May occur with or without associated cervical fractures and may result in dislocations without associated fractures.

Sx: Neck pain or stiffness with attempts at extension or flexion.

Signs: Neck pain exacerbated by extension or flexion. May or may not have neurologic deficiencies noted. Neurologic findings can vary from weakness to quadriplegia. The presence of bilateral symptoms or lower extremity involvement suggests unstable cervical spine injury.

Crs: Depends on degree of injury.

Cmplc: Varying degrees of neurologic dysfunction from mild weakness to complete quadriplegia. Can cause catastrophic neurologic injury. Muscle spasm may mask abnormal motion.

Diff Dx: Cervical strain (see 4.1), cervical spondylosis (see 4.2), cervical fracture.

X-ray:
- A basic 3-view series cervical radiograph should be obtained.
- If radiographs are normal, flexion and extension views should be obtained. Abnormality is indicated by >3.5-mm horizontal displacement with adjacent vertebrae or 11° rotational difference.
- The athlete should actively flex and extend for these views as tolerated and limited by discomfort or symptoms. Pain or neurologic findings limit degree of motion when obtaining these views.
- Athletes that are not alert and oriented should not undergo this examination. Rather, they should be immobilized in a cervical collar until mentation is clear.

Rx: Neurosurgical or orthopedic spine consultation for management options.

Return to Activity: Absolute contraindication to contact or collision activities.

Chapter 5

Shoulder Injuries

Acute Injuries

5.1 Acromioclavicular Separation

Prim Care 2004;31:857; Clin Sports Med 2004;22:387; Phy
    Sportsmed 2001;29:31; Arch Fam Med 1997;6:376; Med Sci
    Sports Exerc 1998;30:S26

Cause: Fall or direct trauma.

Epidem: Common injury in tackling sports (football, soccer, rugby) or
wrestling.

Pathophys: Tearing of acromioclavicular joint capsule and/or coraco-
clavicular ligaments (lateral conoid and medial trapezoid).

Classification:

Grade 1: AC pain without separation; no ligament disruption.

Grade 2: Mild separation; AC joint capsule torn, but coracocla-
vicular ligaments intact.

Grade 3: Severe separation; AC joint capsule and coracoclavi-
cular ligaments torn.

Grade 4: Grade 3 tear of ligaments with distal clavicle posteriorly
displaced into the trapezius.

Grade 5: Grade 3 with severe upward displacement of the distal
clavicle.

Grade 6: Grade 3 with the distal clavicle inferiorly displaced and
trapped under the coracoid.

Sx: Fall on shoulder with arm adducted (at side); pain in the AC area with or without deformity.

Si: Tenderness and soft-tissue swelling over the AC joint with or without deformity positive cross arm test.
- Cross arm test: Patient standing or sitting, arm elevated 90° and internally rotated 90°, examiner forces the arm across the chest (adduction):

   Positive Test = pain isolated to the AC joint

Crs: Self-limiting pain with residual deformity.

Cmplc: Stinger/Burner (see 4.4), clavicle fracture (see 5.2), rotator cuff tear (see 5.4), AC OA (see 5.5), suprascapular nerve injury.

Diff Dx: Clavicle fracture (see 5.2), coracoid fracture, rotator cuff tear (see 5.4), shoulder dislocation (see 5.3), AC OA (see 5.5).

Lab: Consider EMG if suspicious for nerve injury.

X-ray: May be done with or without suspended weights on the arm, rule out coexisting fracture.

Rx:
- Initial: ice, pain medications (NSAID and narcotics), sling for comfort.
- Start pendulum ROM activities as early as pain will allow.
- Shoulder rehab as pain resolves.
- Referral to orthopedics for Grade 4, 5, and 6 injuries, fracture of distal or medial third clavicle or humerus, or patient unwilling to accept cosmetic deformity.
- Referral to physical therapy for rehabilitation pain modalities in acute and early recovery period. See 22.1 for rehab exercises.

Return to Activity: Full ROM without pain; should be able to perform push-ups without pain—Grade 1: 1-2 wk, Grade 2: 3-4 wk, Grade 3: 4-6 wk.

5.2   Clavicle Fracture

Phy Sportsmed 2003;31:30; Phy Sportsmed 1999;27:119; Arch Fam
Med 1997;6:376; Clin Orthop 1989;245:89

Cause: Fall onto shoulder with arm at side (adducted) or direct blow.

Epidem:
- Common in tackling sports—football, soccer, rugby.
- 1:20 in all fractures.
- 44% of shoulder injuries.
- 25% related to athletic activities.

Pathophys:
- 80% fractures are the middle third
- Distal $^1/_2$ 12-15%
- Medial $^1/_3$ rare

Sx: Fall on shoulder or struck by object, audible pop with pain, deformity, and crepitus.

Si: Loss of motion, gross deformity of clavicle, palpable crepitus, r/o
upper extremity neurovascular injury (Brachial Plexus).

Crs: Usually benign in middle third fractures; lateral and medial third
fractures with high complication rate.

Cmplc: Brachial plexus injury, delayed or nonunion, open fracture,
deformity.

Diff Dx: Grade 3-6 AC sprain with significant clavicular displacement
(see 5.1), stinger/burner (see 4.4), coracoid fracture, acromial
fracture, sternoclavicular joint subluxation.

X-ray: classify fracture as medial/lateral/mid third fracture.

Rx:
- Figure-of-eight brace for 4-6 wk.
- Pain control (NSAIDs and narcotics).
- Shoulder ROM as tolerated early (pendulum exercises).
- Rehab, as pain improves.

SHOULDER INJURIES

- Full activity 6 wk (contact sports 8-12 wk), good strength and full ROM.
- Referral to orthopedics for proximal or distal third fractures, non-union, evidence of neurovascular injury, patient unwilling to accept cosmetic deformity.

Return to Activity: At least 6 wk of rest/immobilization; pain-free ROM, and 85% RC strength; normal neuro exam of UE.

5.3 Anterior Shoulder Dislocation

Ortho Clin North Am 2002;33:479; Phy Sportsmed 2002;30:41; Arch Fam Med 1997;6:376; Clin Sports Med 1997;16:669; Orthopedic Sports Med. Philadelphia WB Saunders 1994:580

Cause: Fall or direct blow to shoulder.

Epidem: Anterior dislocation occurs 95% of the time and will be the focus of this discussion; posterior dislocations associated with trauma or seizure; M>F.

Pathopys: The size of the glenoid and humeral head and ROM of the shoulder make it inherently unstable; tear of inferior and middle glenohumeral ligaments and tear or stretch of anterior joint capsule; the "dislocating position" is abduction and external rotation.

Sx: Fall onto or blow to arm that is abducted and externally rotated; h/o prior dislocation.

Si: Arm usually held at side adducted and internally rotated; may see or palpate a large infraacromial sulcus; check distal pulses; check neuro status, especially the sensory distribution of the axillary nerve (posterior deltoid area sensation).

Crs: After reduction age <30 with >80% chance of recurrent dislocation; risk of recurrent dislocation in the >40 y/o group is low; it is common to have rotator cuff tears with older patients.

Cmplc: Instability (recurrent dislocation) (see 5.6); Bankart lesion; adhesive capsulitis (see 5.8); axillary nerve injury; Hill-Sachs lesion; missed diagnosis; unable to reduce.

Diff Dx: Humeral fracture, rotator cuff tear (see 5.4), impingement (see 5.7), deltoid strain, biceps tendon subluxation, posterior dislocation.

X-ray:
- AP and LAT to r/o fracture (may not dx dislocation with these views).
- Axillary or scapular Y view to dx dislocation:
  - Scapular "Y" is a lateral x-ray of the shoulder with the arms of the Y formed by the lateral view of the scapular body, and the wings or upper arms by the scapular spine posteriorly and the coracoid anteriorly; the glenoid with the overlying humeral head will be in the center.
- r/o Bankart lesion: glenoid avulsion fracture from the joint capsule being pulled off seen best in axillary or scapular Y views (it is possible to have a soft tissue Bankart which cannot be see on x-ray).
- r/o Hill-Sachs lesion: posterior humeral head depression from local avascular necrosis due to single or multiple dislocations, seen best with Stryker Notch or axillary views.

Rx:
- Reduction
  1. Rockwood technique or traction/countertraction
     Countertraction with a towel or strap in the axilla and supported by assistant across the table; gentle traction with internal and external rotation; traction may be made easier by a strap or towel around waist and the patient's elbow flexed to 90° then lean back to provide gentle traction.
  2. Stimson technique or "Hang" method
     Hang 10-15 lb from arm with patient prone and arm hanging over edge of table; weight should be taped or

strapped to the arm; if the patient holds the weight, it may increase extremity muscle tone and hinder reduction; leave patient hanging over edge of table undisturbed for 20 min.
3. Self-reduction
   Usually work better with recurrent dislocators.

- Sedation: IV benzodiazepines (must monitor); 15-20 cc intra-articular lidociane 1%.
- Check x-rays and neurovascular status after reduction: confirm reduction, look for Bankart lesion, eval axillary nerve function.
- Pain control measures, ice and sling immobilization.
- Immobilization for short time based on pain (1-2 wk).
- Even shorter immobilization for older patients.
- Begin rehab to strengthen RC as soon as possible; work on isometrics then isotonics (see section 5.4); motion and rehab in frontal plain or across chest is fine; avoid the abducted/externally rotated position (throwing position).
- Referral to orthopedics for inability to reduce, patient <35 y/o (greater chance of repeat dislocation), fracture (humerus, distal clavicle, or Bankart), or recurrent dislocation.

Return to Activity: Full, pain-free ROM and normal rotator cuff (RC) strength; negative instability tests (esp AAT, see 5.6).

5.4   Rotator Cuff Tear

Prim Care 2004;31:789; Arch Fam Med 1997;6:376; J Bone Joint Surg 1989;71-A:499; Am Fam Phys 1996;54:127

Cause: Fall onto shoulder or acute eccentric strain with lift.

Epidem: More common in the >50 y/o population presenting with shoulder pain.

Pathophys:
- Functional Anatomy — RC = **SITS** muscles.
     SITS = **S**upraspinatus (SS), **I**nfraspinatus, **T**eres Minor, **S**ubscapularis.

Then tendons of these muscles form a continuous hood over the humeral head; the SS is the major initiator of abduction and the infraspinatus and teres minor are external rotators (ER).

- The RC functions as humeral depressor to keep humeral head in glenoid as power muscles (deltoid, pectoralis major, latissimus dorsi, teres major) move the arm in gross motions.
- Weakness and degeneration of the RC (from disuse or sport/occupational overuse) allows upward movement of the humeral head imping the RC and bursa between the humeral head and acromion.
- Degeneration and tearing of the RC occurs in may asymptomatic pts as they age and remain active; symptoms more related to "volume" of the tear ie, the size of the hole in the tendon.

Sx: History of a fall or lift causing a significant increase in pain and weakness; usually in the dominant arm; h/o shoulder pain with overhead motion of short or long duration; h/o frequent overhead activities.

Si: Limited motion from weakness or pain; tenderness over anterior rotator cuff (shoulder) area; weak supraspinatus and external rotators; positive impingement signs; may have a positive drop arm test.

- **Drop arm test:**
  Patient standing; full abduct the shoulder then have the patient slowly lower the arm.

  Positive test = arm suddenly drops to side at about 90° abduction or inability to hold the arm at 90° abduction with minimal downward force applied by the examiner.

- **Supraspinatus** (empty can test) (Figure 5.1)
  Shoulder abducted 90°, forward flexed 30°, and internally rotated (thumbs down); patient resists downward direct force; compare to opposite side.

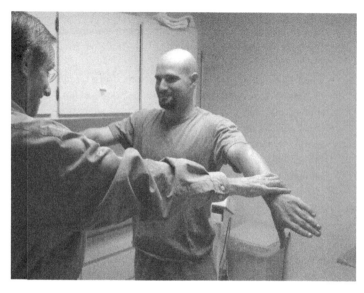

Figure 5.1 Supraspinatus Strength Testing

- **External rotation** (teres minor and infraspinatus):
  Arm at side and elbow flexed to 90°; patient resists inward
      directed force; compare sides.
- **Internal rotation** (subscapularis, pectoralis major, latissimus
  dorsi, teres major):
  Shoulder neutral and elbow flexed to 90°; patient resists out-
      ward direct force; hard to isolate the subscap.
- Subscapularis **lift-off:**
  Arm maximally internally rotated with back of palm resting in
      the lower lumbar area; pt attempts to lift the palm of the
      hand out away from the back against resistance; compare
      to opposite presumed normal side.

- **Bear hug** (Subscap Test): (Phy Sportsmed 2004;32:19)
  Patient places palm of affected arm on opposite shoulder.
     Examiner attempts to displace the palm anteriorly while
     the patient resists. Positive test indicated by inability to
     hold the palm on the opposite shoulder or weakness as
     compared to the opposite side.
- **Impingement test** (Figure 5.2)
  Perform Neer and Hawkin's Impingement signs (see 5.7) after
     subacromial injections of lidocaine (see 1.8); if pain
     relieved but patient still has significant weakness this is
     suggestive of a tear.

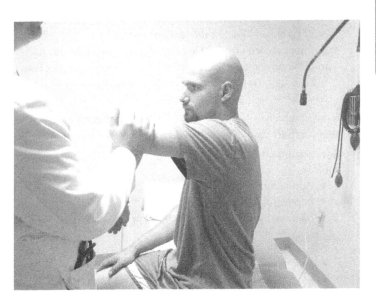

Figure 5.2 Hawkin's Impingement Sign

Crs: Course depends on the arm dominance, functional activity of the pt (occupation, recreation, hobbies), and the volume of the tear (size of the hole in the tendon).

Cmplc: Adhesive capsulitis, glenohumeral OA, nonrepairable tear, chronic pain, and disability.

Diff Dx: Rotator cuff tendinopathy (see 5.9), impingement syndrome (see 5.7), glenohumeral OA, AC OA (see 5.5), C5 or C6 neuropathy/radiculopathy (see 4.3), biceps tendonitis (see 5.10).

X-ray:
- Plain films usually normal, but may demonstrate arthritis or spurring of the AC or GH joints.
- MRI is not the initial study of choice; must correlate findings with the clinical exam; may demonstrate rotator cuff tendinosis (increase signal in the tendon) or tear.
- Arthrogram demonstrates leakage of intra-articular contrast into the subacromial space and will be positive in cases of tear, but cannot quantitate the size of the tear or diagnose tendinosis.

Rx: Rotator cuff rehab 1-4 months (see 22.1); pain control medications; activity modification; consider subacromial injection.

Shoulder rehabilitation:
- Goals
  - Pain reduction
  - Improve range of motion
  - Improved strength for ADLs, sport or occupational activities
- Pain control:
  - Ice (15 min every 2 hr for 24-48 hr)
  - Modalities: high-voltage electrical stimulation, iontophoresis, phonophoresis, TENS
  - Medications: NSAIDs, Tylenol, narcotics
- Motion:
  - Wall climbs

- Pendulum exercises
- Strengthening:
  - Isometric (muscle contraction without motion)—early in rehab when pain more severe (abduction, ER, FF)
  - Isotonic resistance exercise—free weights (3-5 lb) and weight machines, theraband/tubex (surgical tubing)
  - Referral to orthopedics for significant weakness/tear (positive drop arm test), refractory pain and dysfunction/disability, poor response to rehab and observation period (usually >6 months, pt unwilling to accept limitations or disability.

Return to Activity: Pain-free ROM and 85% strength; may need permanent activity, technique, or equipment modifications.

Subacute Injuries

5.5 Acromioclavicular Osteoarthritis

Prim Care 2004;31:857; Am J Phys Med Rehabil 2004;83:791; Arch Fam Med 1997;6:376; Orthopedic Sports Med. Philadelphia: WB Saunders 1994:541

Cause: Repetitive injury (acute and/or chronic).

Epidem:
- Commonly found on shoulder radiographs although most such AC joints are "noisy," but asymptomatic.
- RR 4.6 on right and 2.8 on left for a lifetime of sport activity exceeding 8399 hrs and 12.5 on right and 6.7 on left for high sport activity and high exposure to lifting loads at work (BMJ 1993;27:125).

Pathophys: Chronic overload of joint from overhead/throwing activity and bench press as in weight lifting.

Sx: Shoulder pain with overhead activities; h/o AC separation or activities with frequent blows to the shoulder or weight lifting.

Si: Painful crepitus of AC joint with overhead motion; positive cross-chest adduction test with pain isolated to AC joint.

Crs: Recurrent and unremitting pain with continued activity.

Diff Dx: Osteoid osteoma, undiagnosed clavicle fx (see 5.2), neuralgia from C5 or C6 radiculopathy (see 4.3).

Cmplc: Subacromial impingement and rotator cuff tendinopathy.

X-ray: AC joint narrowing with spurring and osteolysis of distal clavicle.

Rx:

- Symptomatic/pain control.
- Activity modification when symptomatic to reduce or avoid overhead activities, weight lifting, or push-ups.
- Trial of 1-2 cortisone injections into the AC joint 6-8 wk apart (see 1.10 for technique).
- Referral for refractory pain, unwilling/unable to accept activity restrictions, poor response to injections.

Return to Activity: Relative pain-free ROM; functionally can do push-ups without significant pain.

5.6   Shoulder Instability

Prim Care 2004;31:867; Arch Fam Med 1997;6:376; Clin Sports Med 1995;14:761; Clin J Sp Med 1996;6:40

Cause: Congenital ligament laxity or prior dislocation.

Epidem: More common in the younger (<30 y/o) pt presenting with shoulder pain; most common sports include swimming, tennis, baseball, wrestling, and gymnastics.

Pathpohys: Stretched or torn anterior joint capsule and inf and middle glenohumeral ligaments or increased elastin content allowing laxity of multiple joint capsules in the body.

Sx: Recurrent shoulder pain on the overhead active patient; sense of shoulder "going out"; throwers may complain of "dead arm" symptoms (arm goes dead or numb with a hard throw); h/o prior dislocation.

Si: May or may not have painful ROM; may or may not have impingement; weakness of supraspinatus and external rotators; positive instability tests (positive anterior apprehension test and relocation test is most common); if two or three of three instability tests are positive check the other shoulder and other joints for laxity.

Instability tests:
- Anterior Apprehension Test (AAT) (Figure 5.3)
  1. Patient supine at edge of exam table.
  2. Abduct shoulder to 90° and externally rotate at the elbow

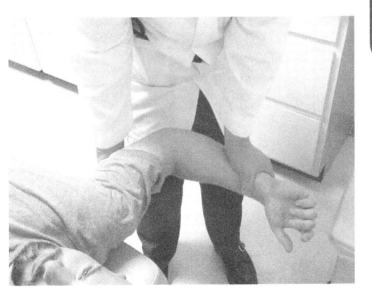

Figure 5.3 Anterior Apprehension Test

while the second hand pushes up (anterior force) on the proximal humerus.
3. **Positive test** = pain or apprehension indicating a sensation of the shoulder going out or reproducing symptoms.
- Relocation test (Figure 5.4):
  1. Follow the AAT with the Relocation test.
  2. Patient supine at edge of table.
  3. Abduct shoulder to 90° and externally rotate at the elbow while the second hand pushes down (posterior force).
  4. **Positive test** = increased tolerance of the external rotation with less or no apprehension.
  5. Anterior instability is confirmed by a positive AAT and relocation test. Positive AAT and negative relocation test may be seen in cases of adhesive capsulitis, rotator cuff tendinosis or tear, and glenohumeral arthritis.

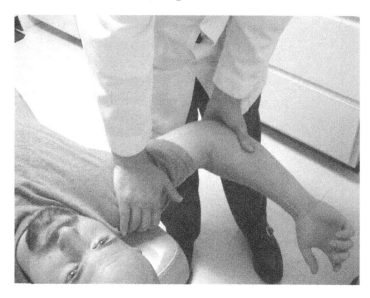

Figure 5.4 Relocation test

- Posterior slide or posterior dislocation test (PDT)
  1. Patient supine at edge of exam table.
  2. Arm abducted 90° and examiner holding wrist while patient relaxes arm.
  3. Examiner applies posterior force on proximal humerus while pulling anteriorly on the wrist, trying to lever the humeral head off the glenoid posteriorly.
  4. **Positive test** = pain or palpation of a posterior subluxed humeral head or a clunk.
- Sulcus sign/inferior dislocation test (IDT) (Figure 5.5):
  1. Patient sitting or supine with the arm at the side.
  2. Apply axial traction on the arm and observe the infra-acromial space.

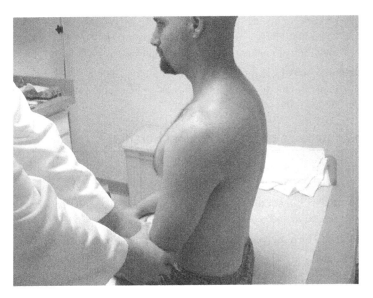

Figure 5.5 Sulcus Sign

3. **Positive test** = dimpling indicating inferior displacement of the humeral head and increased acromial-humeral space. This can be quantitated in cm or grade mild, moderate, and severe and should be compared to the opposite shoulder.

Crs: Progressive of continued symptoms with high-level sport participation.

Cmplc: Hill-Sachs lesion, GOA, thoracic outlet syndrome.

Diff Dx: Rotator cuff tendinopathy or tear (see 5.9 and 5.4), labral tear (see 5.11), humeral tumor or cyst.

X-ray: AP, LAT, and Y or axillary view to r/o glenohumeral arthritis, Hill-Sachs (see 6.3), or Bankart lesions (see 5.3); make sure you order the axillary or Y view.

Rx: Rotator cuff rehabilitation; activity modification until strong or less symptomatic (avoid threatening positions, ie, change sport or profile).

Referral for recurrent symptoms despite rehab or pt unwilling or unable to accept limitations.

Return to Activity: Eighty-five percent strength and pain-free ROM; may need modifications of technique or level of intensity to function without pain.

5.7 Impingement/Subacromial Bursitis

Prim Care 2004;31:789; Arch Fam Med 1997;6:376; Med Sci Sports Exerc 1998;30:S12

Cause: Pinching of rotator cuff (RC) and subacromial bursa between acromion and greater tuberosity with abduction.

Epidem: The most common presentation of primary care shoulder pain.

Pathophys:

- The RC functions as humeral depressor to keep humeral head in glenoid as power muscles (deltoid, pectoralis major, teres major, latissimus dorsi) move the arm in gross motions.

- Weakness and degeneration of the RC (from disuse or sport/occupational overuse) allows upward movement of the humeral head impinging the RC and bursa between the humeral head and acromion.
- Additional risk factors related to acromial shape (Type I: straight and no risk; Type II: semi curved and mod risk; Type III: hooked and high risk), and presence of AC joint spurring from OA with an inferior spur in the subacromial space.

Sx: Superior or lateral sharp shoulder pain with overhead activity; may or may not have had prior pain and subacromial injections; usually in the dominant arm; may have night pain.

Si: Motion may be limited by pain; AC or subacromial crepitus; positive impingement signs (Neer and Hawkin's) (see Figure 5.2); positive impingement test (diagnostic injection) (see 1.8); assess strength of supraspinatus and external rotators; r/o coexistent rotator cuff pathology.

Special tests:
- Neer impingement sign:
  1. Patient standing with arm resting at side.
  2. Examiner internally rotates and forward flexes (elevates) attempting to reach 180°.
  3. **Positive test** = pain usually noted around 120°.
- Hawkin's Impingement Sign (see Figure 5.2):
  1. Patient standing or seated with arm forward flexed to 90°, internally rotated 90° with the elbow flexed 90°.
  2. The examiner attempts to further internally rotate the shoulder driving the greater tuberosity into the acromion.
  3. **Positive test** = pain.
- Impingement test (diagnostic injection) (see 1.8):
  1. Perform impingement signs.
  2. Inject 10 cc of lidocaine 1 or 2% w/o epi
  3. Repeat the impingement signs (Neer and Hawkin's) after 5 min.
  4. **Positive test** = > 50% reduction in pain.

Crs: Recurrent episodes common without adequate RC rehab and continued overuse.

Cmplc: Chronic pain, RC tear.

Diff Dx: RC tear (see 5.4), RC tendinopathy (see 5.9), calcific bursitis (see 5.12), cervical radiculopathy (see 4.4), biceps tendonitis (see 5.10).

X-ray: r/o AC arthritis with spurring on the underside of the AC joint or acromion; r/o subacromial calcifications.

Rx: Activity modification to reduce overhead work; NSAIDs; rotator cuff rehabilitation to focus on strengthening and posterior capsular stretching (see Appendix); trial of subacromial steroid injection. See Section 1.8.

Referral for significant spurring of the AC or subacromial area, refractory symptoms, or suspicion of rotator cuff tear.

Return to Activity: Relatively pain-free ROM and 85% strength; may need prolonged recreational or occupational activity restrictions.

5.8 Adhesive Capsulitis (Frozen Shoulder)

Fed Pract 2003;20:11; Phy Sportsmed 2000;28:23; Arch Fam Med 1997;6:376; Med Sci Sports Exerc 1998;30:S33

Cause: Injury, postop, or idiopathic.

Epidem: Overall incidence in general population 2-5%; females 70% of cases; usually 40-70 y/o pt; 15% will develop sx in opposite shoulder; high incidence in diabetics (10-20%) and more common in pts with h/o hyper and hypothyroidism, diabetes, cardiac disease or cardiac surgery (Phy Sportsmed 2000;28:23).

Pathophys: Joint capsule contracture and subacromial and glenohumeral joint adhesions.

Sx: Painful loss of shoulder motion.

Si: Limited glenohumeral motion with abduction or forward flexion; very limited Apley's; check active ROM first and follow with passive ROM if not full; range of motion should be compared to the opposite noninjured shoulder; exaggerated scapulothoracic motion for abduction; symptoms generally severe enough that impingement, strength, and instability test cannot be performed.

Normal ROM:

Forward flexion (elevation)	0-180°
Abduction	0-180°
External rotation	45°
Internal rotation	55°
Extension	45°

Apley Scratch Test (Figure 5.6) is a functional assessment of the ROM:

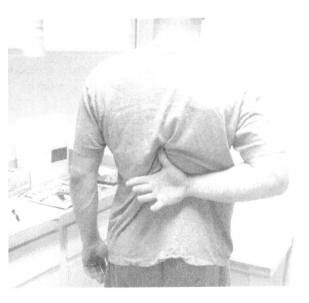

Figure 5.6 Apley test from below

- Apley from below: the patient attempts to scratch between the scapulae from below. This tests adduction and int rotation and can be quantitated by the spinal level reached (T_7: inf angle of scapula, T_3: spine of scapula, T_2: superior angle of the scapula) or compared to the opposite shoulder.
- Apley from above tests abduction and external rotation which can also be quantitated.

Crs: Usually will "thaw out" with time.

Cmplc: Permanent loss of motion, RC tear.

Diff Dx: Glenohumeral OA, RC tear (see 5.4), RC tendinopathy (see 5.9), undiagnosed posterior dislocation, and proximal humeral fracture.

X-ray: r/o AC or glenohumeral arthritis or heterotopic calcifications; MRI may need to be performed to r/o rotator cuff tear.

Rx: The natural history of these shoulders is to improve over time (6-18 months); rotator cuff rehab and formal physical therapy to increase motion; trial of subacromial injection.

Referral for evidence of rotator cuff tear, refractory symptoms after 4-6 months of formal therapy, or evidence of heterotopic calcifications.

Return to Activity: Most pts are functional when they can reach the midlumbar area with the Apley maneuver; pts should have a relative pain-free ROM and 85% supraspinatus strength.

5.9 Rotator Cuff Tendinopathy (Tendinosis)

Clin Sports Med 2003;22:791; Arch Fam Med 1997;6:376; Clin Sports Med Oct 1997;16:674; J Am Acad Orthop Sug 1999;7:32

Cause: Overuse (recreational or occupational).

Epidem: Common cause of shoulder pan in the middle-aged athlete (30-50 y/o); esp if involved in overhead activities.

Pathophys: Chronic overuse with tendon degeneration and dysfunction; microscopic exam of tendon demonstrates disorganized fibroblasts (angiofibroblastic dysplasia—see pathophys in 6.1).

Sx: Shoulder pain with overhead motion of short or long duration; h/o frequent overhead activities; may have a history of a fall causing a significant increase in pain and weakness; usually in the dominant arm.

Si: Limited motion from weakness or pain; tenderness over anterior rotator cuff (shoulder) area; weak supraspinatus and external rotators; positive impingement signs; in cases of tears impingement test may relieve pain but patient still has significant weakness.

Crs: Progressive dysfunction with recurrent pain episodes/exacerbations.

Cmplc: Adhesive capsulitis, RC tear, calcific tendonitis.

Diff Dx: Adhesive capsulitis (see 5.8), RC tear (see 5.4), impingement (see 5.7), AC OA (see 5.5).

X-ray: Usually normal, but may demonstrate arthritis or spurring of AC joint, calcific tendonitis or bursitis, or glenohumeral OA; MRI is not the initial study of choice; must correlate findings with the clinical exam; may demonstrate rotator cuff tendinosis (increase signal in the tendon) or tear.

Rx:
- Rotator cuff rehab 1-4 months (see 22.1).
- Pain control measures:
  - NSAIDs, ice after activity, and prn narcotics.
- Activity modification.
- Consider subacromial injection to buy some pain relief to allow pt to continue with rehab.

- Referral for refractory pain, poor response to good organized rehab >4-6 months, evidence of tear, unwilling to accept limitations or disability.

Return to Activity: Pain-free ROM without impingement and 85% RC strength (supraspinatus and external rotators).

5.10 Biceps Tendinitis

Phys Med Rehabil Clin N Am 2004;15:511; Arch Fam Med 1997;6:376; Phy Sportsmed 1999;27:95

Cause: Biceps tendon inflammation or subluxation out of the intertubercular groove.

Epidem: Often associated with RC tear or tendinosis.

Pathophys: The long head of the biceps assists the rotator cuff as a shoulder depressor and dynamic stabilizer; it passes between the greater and lesser tuberosities in the intertubercular groove and becomes an intra-articular tendon inserting into the superior glenoid.

Sx: H/o overuse throwing or other overhead activities; similar to rotator cuff tendinosis; pain with overhead motion or shoulder elevation against resistance.

Si: Anterior shoulder pain; with external rotation the long head in the intertubercular groove can be palpated to be tender.

Speed's Test (Figure 5.7):
- Test for subluxation or tendinitis of the biceps tendon.
- Patient standing and both arms forward flexed 60° in neutral rotation (thumbs up).
- Examiner applies a downward force while the patient resists.
- **Positive test** = pain or giving way (weakness without pain may be noted in old biceps ruptures).

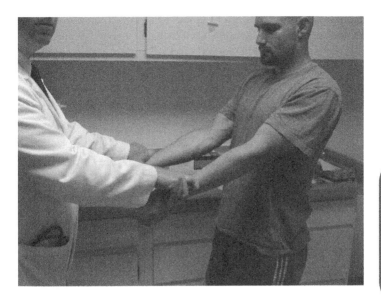

Figure 5.7 Speed's Test

Yergason's Test:
- Tests subluxation of the biceps tendon.
- Patient standing with arm at side and elbow flexed to 90° and forearm neutral (thumb up).
- Patient resists as the examiner extends the elbow and pronates the forearm.
- **Positive test** = pain or pop in the biceps tendon.

Crs: Chronic pain with overhead motion.

Cmplc: Rupture.

Diff Dx: RC tear/tendinopathy (see 5.4 and 5.9), calcific bursitis (see 5.12).

X-ray: Usually normal.

Rx: Relative rest from overhead and heavy lifting activities; consider physical therapy modalities for local pain relief; biceps and rotator cuff strengthening; consider local corticosteroid injection. Referral for refractory pain with rotator cuff dysfunction, evidence of acute or chronic rupture.

Return to Activity: Pain-free ROM and 85% strength; negative Speed's test.

5.11 Labral Tear

Prim Care 2004;31:867; Prim Care 2004;31:831; Arch Fam Med 1997;6:376; Am J Sports Med 1996;24:721; Clin Sports Med 2000;19:115; Phy Sportsmed 1999;27:73

Cause: Dislocation, fall, and weight lifting injury.

Epidem: Common in the younger pt with instability.

Pathophys:
- The labrum is a redundancy of the joint capsule as it attaches to the glenoid that increases the contact area for the humeral head to improve stability.
- Tears usually traumatic: Number one violent eccentric load on the biceps tendon avulsing it superiorly creating the SLAP lesion (Superior Labral Anterior Posterior); number two the humeral head levers on anterior or posterior labrum with ROM.
- If there is a heavy axial load with this motion the labrum may be torn; number three traumatic tear with anterior or posterior dislocation.
- SLAP lesion classification:
  - Type I—frayed edge of superior labrum
  - Type II—detached biceps tendon
  - Type III—bucket handle tearing of superior labrum
  - Type VI—type III with splitting extending into the biceps tendon

Sx: Painful click or pop in shoulder.

Si: Good ROM and usually good strength; no impingement; may have signs of instability (AAT, relocation, PDT, sulcus); positive crank or modified crank; positive "SLAPrehension" test.

Crank Test (Figure 5.8):
- Pt supine with shoulder hanging over edge of table.
- Shoulder abducted to 90°.
- Elbow flexed 90° and examiner provides axial load on humerus as the humerus is rotated (crank).
- **Positive test** = pain with rotation; ± click.

Modified crank test:
- Similar positioning as the Crank test.
- Examiner now provides an axial load/force while the humerus is circumducted pinching the labrum 360°.

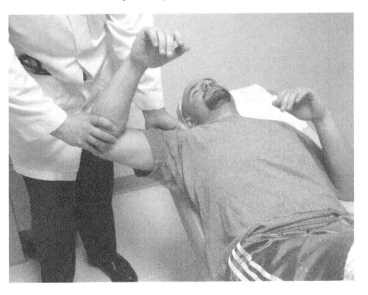

Figure 5.8   Crank Test (Compression Rotation)

- **Positive test** = pain and or click when the affected part of the labrum is pinched; it is usually good to reproduce the symptoms several times for consistency to confirm.

Obrien Test (Figure 5.9)

- Patient sitting with arm elevated 90° and 45° horizontal adduction and maximal internal rotation.
- Examiner resists attempted adduction and forward flexion of the arm.
- **Positive test** = pain or a painful pop.

Crs: Some will become pain free with time.

Cmplc: Instability; accelerated GH OA.

Diff Dx: Loose body, RC tendinopathy or tear (see 5.9 and 5.4).

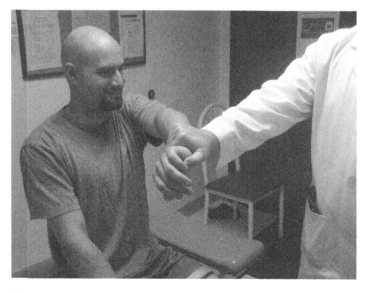

Figure 5.9   Obrien Test (Active Compression)

X-ray: Plain films usually normal or may have Bankart or Hill-Sachs (see 5.3); MRI with contrast will demonstrate labral pathology the best.

Rx:
- RC rehab and observation with activity modification.
- Will have problems similar to the pt with instability.
- Referral for chronic symptoms, chronic instability, SLAP lesions.

Return to Activity: Pain-free ROM and 85% strength; asymptomatic instability tests and Crank and SLAPrehension tests; functional testing of push-ups, throw, and jumping jacks.

5.12 Calcific Bursitis/Tendinitis

Ortho Clin North Am 2003;34:567; Arch Fam Med 1997;6:376; Phy Sportsmed 1999;27:27; Nejm 1999;340:1533

Cause: Calcium deposition in subacromial bursa or rotator cuff tendons.

Epidem: 30-60 y/o pt; 20-30% bilateral; up 20% may be asymptomatic.

Pathophys: Inflammation causing heterotopic calcification that functions as a persistent local irritant or abnormal healing of RC degeneration.

Sx: Subacromial pain.

Si: Impingement signs, rotator cuff dysfunction.

Crs: Usually chronic pain until resolved.

Cmplc: Chronic pain, RC tear.

Diff Dx: RC tendinopathy (see 5.9), subacromial impingement (see 5.7), fracture (greater or lesser tuberosity), tumor.

Rx:
- Usually will need aggressive physical therapy.
- Rotator cuff rehab for ROM and strengthening.

- Subacromial/intralesional steroid injection.
- PT modalities (phonophoresis and US) for mobilization.
- Referral to orthopedics for surgical removal if refractory to conservative management or evidence of tear.

Return to Activity: Pain-free ROM and 85% strength and desire to return.

Chapter 6

Elbow Problems

6.1 Lateral Epicondylitis/Tendinosis (Lateral Tennis Elbow)

J Bone Joint Surg 1999;81-A:259; Clin Sports Med 1992;11:851; Curr Opin Orthop 2003;14:291

Cause: Repetitive or overuse injury of the common extensor mechanism; primarily the extensor carpi radialis brevis (ECRB) and sometimes the extensor digitorum communis (EDC).

Epidem:
- Higher incidence in athletes >35 yr, especially those participating in racquet sports; higher activity level (sports or occupational).
- Poor technique; inadequate fitness level.

Pathophys:
- Repetitive eccentric overload of ECRB and/or the EDC, typically from tennis backhand, leading to degenerative histological changes within the tendon.
- Early reports consistently described this process as inflammatory in nature; however, recent studies have confirmed the presence of fibroblasts, vascular hyperplasia, and disorganized collagen (angiofibroblastic hyperplasia) with a paucity of acute or chronic inflammatory cells, supporting the use of the term "tendinopathy" instead of "tendonitis."

Sx:

- Lateral elbow pain typically with activities.
- Occasional swelling and weakness of wrist extensors.
- Numbness and parasthesias are uncommon.

Si:

- Focal tenderness to palpation of common extensors overlying the lateral epicondyle and extending 1-2 cm distally.
- Typically pain is elicited with resisted wrist extension while the elbow is in full extension, pain with the elbow flexed may indicate more advanced disease.
- Pain may also be elicited with resisted supination.
- Care should be taken to fully examine the shoulder as well, since it is not uncommon to uncover associated rotator cuff weakness.

Crs:

- Initially pain after activities, which is self-remitting.
- Without treatment pain typically progresses to pain during activities only and may begin to affect activities of daily living and eventually become constant as well as disturb sleep.

Cmplc: Persistent overload may lead to irreversible tendon damage and possible rupture.

Diff Dx: Cervical radiculopathy at C6-C7 (see 4.4); posterior interosseous nerve (PIN) entrapment (see 6.4); radial head fracture; fibromyalgia (if multiple other soft-tissue tender points identified); tumor.

X-ray: Calcification or exostosis at the epicondyle or in the tendon close to the tendon attachment may be seen in up to 20% of cases; however, this appears to have no prognostic implications. Ultrasound may show increased blood flow near the lateral epicondyle.

Rx:

Preventive:

- Flexibility: stretching exercises for spine, shoulder (including scapula stabilizers: pectoralis, latissimus, rhomboids, trapezius), arm (biceps, triceps), forearm (wrist flexors and extensors).
- Strength: progressive resistive exercise for the shoulder, elbow, wrist, and grip.
- Proper technique: strike the ball in front of the body with the wrist and elbow extended, allowing the upper arm and torso not the wrist extensors to provide stroke power.
- Equipment: lightweight racquet of low vibration material (graphite, epoxies); appropriate grip size (handle circumference should be equal to the measured distance from the tip of the ring finger to the proximal palmar crease, along its radial border); low string tension.

Therapeutic:

- Protect, rest, ice, compression, elevation, medications, modalities (PRICEMM).
- Rehabilitation exercises to include: stretching of wrist flexors and extensors; strengthening of wrist, elbow, and shoulder muscles especially rotator cuff (see 22.2)
- Modalities to the affected area (ice, heat, ultrasound, electrical stimulation) with the goal of allowing individual to participate in rehabilitation program; general body conditioning.
- Control of force loads as patient returns to activities: counterforce brace (forearm strap); improved sports technique; consider developing a two-handed backhand stroke; control intensity, duration and frequency of activities; appropriate equipment/racquet (see above).
- Consider steroid injection if pain continues to limit participation in rehabilitation program (see 2.7).
- Consider surgery for failure to respond to an appropriate rehabilitation program of 6 months or greater or an unacceptable quality of life.

- Alternative modalities for resistant cases have been investigated and include botulinum toxin A, extracorporal shock wave therapy, acupuncture, and autologous blood injections.

6.2 Medial Epicondylitis / Tendinosis (Golfer's or Pitcher's Elbow)

Am J Sports Med 1994;22:674; Techniques Hand and Upp Extrem Surg 2003;7:190

Cause: Repetitive or overuse injury of the common flexor mechanism: primarily effecting the flexor carpi radialis, pronator teres, flexor carpi ulnaris muscles.

Epidem:
- Higher incidence in athletes >35 yr.
- Golfers, tennis players, and throwing sports.

Pathophys:
- Repetitive eccentric overload of common flexors and pronator teres typically occurring in trail arm during a golf swing, forehand in racquet sports, or throwing arm.
- Degenerative histological changes within the tendon, angiofibroblastic hyperplasia (see 6.1).

Sx:
- Medial elbow pain typically with activities.
- Occasional swelling and weakness of wrist flexors and pronator.
- Numbness and parasthesias are uncommon.

Si:
- Focal tenderness to palpation of over the tip of the medial epicondyle extending distally 1-2 cm.
- Often increased pain with resisted wrist flexion and pronation.
- May also be associated rotator cuff weakness.
- Check for positive Tinel's sign at the cubital tunnel to rule out associated ulnar nerve entrapment (see 15.10).

Crs:
- Initially pain after activities, which is self-remitting; progresses to pain during activities only.
- Without treatment, pain may begin to affect daily living and eventually become constant as well as disturb sleep.

Cmplc: Persistent overload may lead to irreversible tendon damage and possible rupture.

Diff Dx: Ulnar (medial) collateral ligament (UCL) sprain or rupture (see 6.7); cervical radiculopathy at C5-C6 (see 4.4); ulnar nerve entrapment at the elbow (cubital tunnel syndrome) (see 6.3), tumor.

X-ray:
- Calcification or exostosis at the epicondyle or at the tendon attachment.
- Calcification within the UCL, may suggest concomitant instability.

Rx:

Preventive:
- Flexibility: stretching exercises for spine, shoulder (including scapula stabilizers: pectoralis, latissimus, rhomboids, trapezius), arm (biceps, triceps), forearm (wrist flexors and extensors).
- Strength: progressive resistive exercise for the shoulder, elbow, wrist, and grip.
- Proper technique: for racquet sports, see discussion of lateral epicondylitis, 7.1.
- Equipment: for racquet sports see discussion of lateral epicondylitis, 7.1. In golf, clubs of proper weight, length and grip may be selected utilizing the assistance of a golf professional or expert.

Therapeutic:
- Protect, rest, ice, compression, elevation, medications, modalities (PRICEMM).

- Rehabilitation exercises to include: stretching of wrist flexors and extensors; strengthening of wrist, elbow, and shoulder muscles especially rotator cuff; modalities to the affected area (ice, heat, ultrasound, high-voltage galvanic stimulation) with the goal of allowing individual to participate in rehabilitation program.
- General body conditioning.
- Control of force loads as patient returns to activities (counter-force brace; improved sports technique; control intensity, duration, and frequency of activities; appropriate equipment). See 6.1 Rx. Improve the golf swing: ensure the swing plane is not too steep (perpendicular to the ground) or too flat (parallel to the ground). Consider a graphite shaft and larger heads of golf clubs to minimize vibration forces.
- Consider steroid injection and night splinting, if pain continues to limit participation in rehabilitation program.
- Consider surgery for failure to respond to an appropriate rehabilitation program of 6 months or greater or an unacceptable quality of life.

6.3 Posterior Interosseous Nerve (PIN) Entrapment (Supinator Syndrome, Radial Tunnel Syndrome)

Electrodiagnostic Medicine: Lippincott-Ravel Publishing, 2nd ed, Philadelphia, 2002 p 1087; Techniques Hand and Upp Extrem Surg 2002;6:209

Cause:
- Compression of nerve by lipoma, hemangioma, ganglia, fibroma; missile fragment; laceration.
- Fracture and dislocation (Monteggia fracture—proximal ulnar fracture with posterior radial head dislocation).

Epidem:
- Repetitive wrist use.
- Thirty percent of individuals have a sharp fibrous opening of the supinator muscle where the PIN enters.

Pathophys:

Radial Tunnel Syndrome: Entrapment of the radial nerve where it pierces between the brachialis and bracioradialis before entering the supinator.

Supinator Syndrome: Entrapment of the PIN at the *arcade of Frohse* (fibrous opening in the superficial head of the supinator muscle).

Sx: Dull or sharp pain in the extensor muscle mass of the forearm; no sensory loss; weakness of wrist and/or finger extension.

Si:
- Pain with deep palpation along the proximal radius.
- Normal sensory exam, because nerve carries motor fibers.
- Radial deviation with wrist extension because of the preservation of the extensor carpi radialis unopposed by the dennervated extensor carpi ulnaris.
- Weakness and often pain with resisted middle finger extension "Middle finger test."
- Supination should be checked with the elbow at 90° flexion to help remove the biceps. This may reveal pain and/or weakness.

Crs: Severe injury may lead to complete wrist drop.

Cmplc: Without recognition and proper management, irreversible nerve damage may occur.

Diff Dx: Lateral epicondylitis (see 6.1); extensor tenosynovitis; C6-C7 radiculopathy (see 4.4).

Lab: EMG/NCV helpful for identifying location and severity of injury.

X-ray:
- Plain films to rule out fracture or exostosis.
- CT or MRI to rule out possible mass or space occupying lesion.
- Further imaging may also assist with preoperative planning when indicated.

ELBOW PROBLEMS

Rx:

- In the absence of a mass, 8-12 wk of relative rest, anti-inflammatory medications and avoidance of provocative activities should be allowed for spontaneous recovery.
- If mass is identified or failure to resolve spontaneously, surgery is indicated.

6.4   Olecranon Bursitis

J Accid Emerg Med 1996;13:351; Physical Medicine and Rehabilitation, 2nd ed, Philadelphia, WB Saunders 2000, p 810; Phy Sportsmed 2000;28:46

Cause: Direct blow or prolonged pressure over the olecranon.

Epidem:

- One of the most frequently inflamed bursae.
- Common in contact sports and in laborers.
- More common in males aged 30-60 yr.

Pathophys:

- Inflammatory condition resulting from trauma, infection, or other arthropathy.
- Infection typically involves a break of the skin providing a portal of entry of bacteria (*Staphylococcus aureus* representing 90% of cases).
- Permanent damage to the epithelial lining of the bursa predisposes individual to repeated attacks.
- Chronic conditions result in thickening and fibrosis of the bursal lining.

Sx:

- Acute or chronic pain and swelling overlying the olecranon.
- Often presents as an acute traumatic episode superimposed upon a more chronic condition.

Si:

- Palpation of bursal sac reveals tenderness and swelling.
- Infection should be suspected with the presence of erythema and warmth.
- Range of motion is typically not limited unless extreme elbow flexion causes increased skin tension over swollen bursa.
- Fibrous trabeculation within the bursa is often palpated in chronic cases.

Crs: Recurrence is common.

Cmplc: Untreated infectious bursitis may lead to sepsis and serious complications.

Diff Dx: Infection: usually *S. aureus*, less common β-hemolytic streptococci; arthritis: manifestation of rheumatoid arthritis or crystalline arthropathy (such as gout); fracture; cellulitis; tendinitis (esp triceps).

Lab:

- Aspirated fluid should be sent for crystals, cell count, gram stain, and culture.
- Elevated WBC suspicious of infection.
- Uric acid if considering gout.
- Rheumatoid factor if considering RA.

X-ray: Helpful to rule out possible fracture, calcification, tumor.

Rx:

- Aspiration should be performed with an 18-gauge needle, posterior-lateral approach, zig-zag fashion to minimize fistula formation if significant swelling or suspected infections. Fluid should be sent to lab and appropriate antibiotic started, as indicated.
- For noninfectious bursitis, compression and ice packs should be applied for 15-20 min, several times per day during first 2-5 d.

ELBOW PROBLEMS

- Heat may apply particularly after the first 72 hr to hasten fluid absorption.
- Physical therapy modalities (phonophoresis, electrical stimulation) may be helpful for recalcitrant inflammation.
- Elbow pads cushion the region from further trauma.
- NSAIDs can help decrease pain and inflammation.
- Steroid injections should be considered rarely in chronic bursitis as they may cause fat pad atrophy, reducing the natural padding of the olecranon and therefore predispose to recurrent episodes.
- Surgical removal of the bursa may be indicated in severe refractory bursitis. Appropriate padding of the elbow should be incorporated into primary and secondary prevention. Physical therapy should be considered postoperatively for regaining or maintaining range of motion and strength of the elbow.

6.5 Traumatic Elbow Injuries (Sprain, Strain, Fracture)

Phys Sportsmed 1996;24:43; Curr Opin Rheumatol 2002;14:160

Cause:
- Collision.
- Fall on outstretched arm.
- Throwing injury.

Epidem:
- Contact sports.
- Activities at risk of falling (gymnastics, skateboarding).

Pathophys: Bony or soft-tissue overload.

Sx: Acute elbow pain, swelling, reduced range of motion.

Si:
- Careful palpation for focal areas of tenderness.
- Assess for restriction of range of motion (compare to uninjured side).

- Assess for ligamentous stability (ulnar collateral ligament (UCL) stability is checked by applying a valgus stress with the elbow flexed to 20°, radial collateral ligament is checked by applying a varus stress).
- Check for dislocation (usually posterolateral).
- Careful neurovascular examination is imperative.

Crs: Early recognition and treatment of underlying pathology usually resolves without complications.

Cmplc:
- Inappropriate diagnosis and treatment may lead to serious deformity and long-term disability.
- Failure to recognize neurovascular compromise may result in loss of limb.

Diff Dx: Fracture; dislocation; ligamentous sprain.

X-ray:
- Acute injuries warrant prompt imaging. One should obtain anteroposterior, lateral, olecranon, and occasional oblique views.
- *Montaggia fracture:* fracture of the proximal third of the ulna and dislocation of the radial head.

Rx:
- Although gentle elbow flexion and forearm rotation to a neutral position may result in spontaneous reduction of dislocation, it is best to splint the arm and not move it until the patient can be transported to an emergency room where x-rays may be obtained and the reduction may be performed in a controlled environment.
- Immediate reduction may be considered if no medical facility is nearby and neurovascular injury has occurred from fracture or dislocation.
- Traumatic injuries leading to ligamentous disruption, fracture, or dislocation warrant immediate splinting and orthopedic consultation.

ELBOW PROBLEMS

6.6 Medial Collateral Ligament (MCL) Instability

AAOS Instr/course Lect 1999;48:383; Sports Med Arthro Rev
  2003;11:15

Cause: Forceful extension of the elbow, accompanied by a valgus
  stress often created during throwing activities.

Epidem:
- Sudden traumatic event such as in wrestling or javelin
  throwing.
- Repetitive stress in throwing or overhead sports such as during
  the volleyball serve.

Pathophys:
- Acute overload of ligament tensile strength.
- Repetitive stress leads to progressive microscopic damage to
  the MCL, progressing in four stages:
  1. Edema and inflammation
  2. Dissociation of ligamentous fibers
  3. Calcification
  4. Ossification

Sx:
- Pain along the medial elbow during late cocking or accelera-
  tion phases of throwing.
- Athlete may experience "opening" or "giving way" of elbow.
- Ulnar nerve irritation (paresthesias to the ulnar aspect of the
  forearm and hand).

Si:
- Tenderness to palpation along the MCL, particularly 2 cm
  distal to the medial epicondyle.
- Pain and instability when a valgus stress is applied to the elbow
  in 20°-30° of flexion.
- *Milking Maneuver:* performed by pulling on the thumb and pal-
  pating along the medial collateral ligament while the elbow is

flexed, forearm supinated, and shoulder extended. The generation of pain and a sense of laxity (joint line gapping) indicate a positive sign.

Crs: Untreated athletes will typically alter their biomechanics promoting further damage.

Cmplc: Advanced degenerative changes.

Diff Dx: Medial epicondylitis (see 6.2); ulnar nerve entrapment (see 6.3); osteoarthritis.

X-ray: Radiographs will often reveal loose bodies, marginal osteophytes, ligamentous calcifications, or heterotopic bone formation. MRI may help to clarify partial or complete tear of the MCL.

Rx:

Preventive:
- Good throwing mechanics.
- Ensure adequate warm-up.
- Appropriate conditioning (strength training and aerobic conditioning) to resist fatigue.
- Flexibility not only of upper extremities but of trunk, low back, and hamstrings, as well.

Nonsurgical:
- Apply principles of PRICEMM.
  - Rest may need to extend 2 to 4 wk.
- Progress to active range of motion when athlete is pain free.
- Strength training is added shortly thereafter.
- Begin return to throwing program when athlete achieves symmetric range of motion and strength.

Surgical:
- Indications:
  - Acute complete rupture.
  - Chronic pain and/or symptomatic instability that fails to respond to a minimum of 3 mo of adequate rehabilitation.

6.7 Distal Biceps Tendon Injury

J Am Acad Orthop Sug 1999;7:199; Sports Med Arthro Rev 2003;11:47

Cause:
- Usually a single traumatic event results in overload of tendon, causing avulsion of the tendon from its insertion to the radial tuberosity as well as frequently a tear of the bicipital aponeurosis. All reported cases have involved an extension force with the elbow in 90° flexion.

Epidem:
- Dominant extremity of males aged 30-60 yr.
- Mean age 50 yr.
- Weight lifting especially in the presence of anabolic steroid use.

Pathophys:
- Degenerative changes of the tendon over time compromise the structural integrity of the tendon predisposing it to rupture.
- Hypovascularity of the tendon at its insertion has been implicated.
- Spurring of the radial tuberosity is common.
- An intact bicipital aponeurosis (lacertus fibrosus) will prevent proximal migration of the ruptured tendon into the arm.

Sx:
- Sudden sharp, tearing pain in the antecubital fossa or lower anterior aspect of the brachium for the first few hours, then a dull ache persisting for weeks or longer.
- Weakness of elbow flexion, supination, and grip strength.

Si:
- Ecchymosis in the antecubital fossa.
- Immediate swelling and tenderness.
- A visible and palpable defect of the distal biceps muscle is usually obvious in a complete tear.

- Incomplete or partial rupture typically reveals crepitus or grinding with forearm rotation and absence of a palpable defect.
- Significant motion loss is not characteristic.
- Weakness with resisted elbow flexion with the forearm supinated.
- Weakness with resisted supination with the elbow at 90° flexion.

Crs: Early recognition and treatment of underlying pathology usually resolves without complications.

Cmplc: Inappropriate diagnosis and treatment may lead to serious deformity and long-term disability. Failure to recognize neurovascular compromise may result in loss of limb.

Diff Dx: Fracture, dislocation, ligamentous sprain.

X-ray: An MRI is helpful for making or confirming the diagnosis, although not always reliable in distinguishing partial tears from bicipital tendinosus. Routine use in biceps tendon ruptures is not indicated.

Rx:
- Complete tears should be treated with early surgical repair, followed by passive range of motion in 4-5 d, then active flexion and extension and forearm rotation in 7-10 d. Light weights (1-2 lbs) are introduced in 4-6 wk. A patient may expect to return to full activities in 3-6 months, depending on the demands of the sport and progress in rehabilitation phase.
- Partial or incomplete tears may not always require surgery, however, may result in a 30% loss of flexion strength and a 40% loss of supination strength.

ELBOW PROBLEMS

Chapter 7

Hand Injuries

Tendon Injuries

7.1 Mallet Finger

Clin Sports Med 1998;17:449

Cause: Axial load against an actively extending finger.

Epidem:
- Originally described in baseball, but can occur in any activity where the finger is subject to "jamming."
- Frequently missed initially with subsequent deformity and medicolegal consequences.

Pathophys:
- Can result in a dorsal bony avulsion or a grade III (complete disruption) injury to the extensor digitorum tendon.

Sx:
- Pain at the dorsal distal interphalangeal joint.

Si:
- Inability to extend the isolated DIP.
- Tenderness over the dorsal proximal aspect of the distal phalanx.

X-ray:
- Bony avulsion from the dorsal proximal distal phalanx seen in approximately 20-30% of cases.

Rx:
- Initially treated with PRICEMM (Protection, relative rest, ice, compression, elevation, medications, and modalities) and analgesia as needed.
- No avulsion fracture: splint DIP fully extended for 6-8 w straight and an additional 6-8 w, if engaged in athletic activities.
- Bony avulsion with <30% of joint space involved are frequently unstable and require surgical fixation. If stable, dorsal finger splint in full extension for 4 w.
- Bony avulsion with >30% of joint space involved: refer for possible ORIF.
- Permanent DIP extensor lag, if untreated. Watch for pressure necrosis from splint.

Return to Activity:
- May return as soon as can be adequately splinted (as discussed above).

7.2 Jersey Finger (Football Finger)

Clin Sports Med 1998;17:449

Cause: Forced extension of the distal phalanx while actively flexing the DIP (eg, athlete grabbing onto a jersey).

Epidem: Common in football, rugby, martial arts or any sport where grabbing an opponent's clothing can occur.

Pathophys:
- Results in either a grade III tear or a bony avulsion fracture of the flexor digitorum profundus tendon.
- An avulsion fracture of the volar lip of the distal phalanx limits retraction and enables repair by ORIF.
- Pure tendon avulsions may retract to the PIP or palm.
- If retracted to the palm, the blood supply via the vincula brevum and longum is compromised.

Sx: Pain and swelling at the DIP.

Si:

- Unable to flex the isolated DIP with localized tenderness at the level of retraction of the avulsed segment.
- The flexor digitorum profundus is examined by holding the PIP straight and asking the athlete to flex the DIP.
- The superficialis is tested by holding the MCP straight and asking the athlete to flex the PIP.

X-ray: PA, lateral, and oblique views will document an avulsed fragment and may help localize the level of retraction.

Rx:

- Initial treatment is PRICEMM and analgesics, as needed.
- Refer for surgical repair within 3 w with retraction to PIP, within 1 w if retracted to the palm.

Return to Activity: 6-12 w following surgery, depending on chosen sport.

7.3 Traumatic Dislocation of the Extensor Hood (Boxer's Knuckle)

Clin Sports Med 1998;17:449

Cause: Caused by direct blow to the flexed MCP or by flexion and ulnar deviation force across the MCP.

Epidem: Collision or contact sports.

Pathophys: Disruption of the sagittal fibers (usually radial) allowing the extensor tendon to sublux off the apex of the MCP into the valley between the MC heads.

Sx: Pain and swelling over the dorsum of the MCP.

Si:

- MCP is tender dorsally with inability to actively extend the MCP joint from a flexed position.
- After passive extension of the joint, the patient is able to maintain extension.

X-ray: Plain radiographs usually normal.

Rx:

- Initially treated with PRICEMM, splinting, and analgesics as needed.
- Splint the MCP in full extension with the PIP free for 4 w.
- Active ROM exercises are begun at 4 w with the splint worn at all other times.
- Splint is discontinued at 8 w.
- Old injuries should be referred for possible surgical correction.

7.4 Central Slip Avulsion

Clin Sports Med 1998;17:449

Cause: Volar directed force on the middle phalanx against a semi-flexed finger attempting to extend.

Epidem: Contact and collision sports.

Pathophys: Disruption of the central slip of the extensor digitorum communis tendon over the PIP joint allowing for migration of the lateral bands volar to the axis of the joint ("Boutonniere" deformity).

Sx: Pain and swelling over the PIP joint.

Si:

- The PIP is in 15-30° of flexion with point tenderness over the dorsal lip of the middle phalanx.
- There is an inability to actively extend the PIP.

X-ray: May show an avulsion fracture at the dorsal base of the middle phalanx.

Rx:
- Initially treated with PRICEMM as needed.
- PIP is splinted in full extension for 4-5 w and further protected during sporting activity for an additional 6-8 w.
- While splinted the DIP should be allowed to flex to help relocate the lateral bands back to their normal position.
- If an avulsion fragment involves >⅓ of the joint, they should be referred for possible ORIF.

Return to Activity: 4-8 w depending on chosen activity.

7.5 Trigger Finger

Clin Sports Med 1998;17:449

Cause: Nonspecific flexor tenosynovitis from overdemand.

Epidem: Rowing, rock climbing, or any activity requiring repetitive finger flexion.

Pathophys: Most common in the flexor tendons of the thumb, middle, and long fingers.

Sx: Difficulty straightening involved finger (triggering), especially in AM, variable degree of pain.

Si: Variable amount of tenderness over flexor tendon sheath aggravated by active finger flexion or passive extension. Palpable nodule in flexor tendon sheath.

X-ray: Radiographs not indicated.

Rx:
- Early or no triggering: splint finger at night.
- Triggering: inject flexor tendon sheath through a mid-lateral approach over distal ⅓ of the proximal phalanx. Repeat in 6-8 w, if symptoms persist (max 2 injections and consider ortho referral). Splint at night.

Return to Activity: As symptoms allow.

Ligament Injuries

7.6   Collateral Ligament Tears

Clin Sports Med 1986;5:757

Cause: Result from valgus or varus stress to the PIP, DIP, or MCP.

Epidem: Collision and contact sports.

Pathophys: Causes partial or complete tears of the ulnar or radial collateral ligaments.

Sx: Pain and swelling at the involved joint.

Si: Laxity with valgus or varus stress. The joint may be stable or unstable with active flexion and extension.

X-ray: May show avulsion fracture from capsular insertion.

Rx:
- Initially treated with PRICEMM, splinting, and analgesics as needed.
- Stable with active ROM: buddy tape finger to finger adjacent to side of injury for 3 w.
- Unstable with active ROM or obvious angulation: refer for possible surgical repair.

Return to Activity:
- As symptoms allow, with protective splinting.

7.7   PIP Volar Plate Rupture (without Dislocation)

Clin Sports Med 1986;5:757

Cause: Hyperextension injury causing the distal portion of the volar plate to rupture from its attachment to the middle phalanx.

Epidem: Common in volleyball, football, or any sport where the finger is subject to hyperextension.

Pathophys: The loss of the volar stabilizing force of the PIP allows the extensor tendon to gradually pull the PIP into a hyperextension deformity (reverse Boutonniere).

Sx: Pain and swelling at the PIPJ.

Si:
- The PIP is in varying degrees of hyperextension with maximal tenderness over the volar aspect of the PIP.
- With active extension and flexion, the hyperextended PIP often "locks" in the extended position with an inability to initiate flexion.

X-ray: PA, lateral, and oblique may show an avulsion fragment at the base of the middle phalanx.

Rx:
- Initially treated with PRICEMM, as needed.
- Extension block splint for 3 w with the PIP blocked at 20-30° of flexion, then buddy tape.

Return to Activity: 3-6 w with protective splint.

7.8 "Skiers" or "Gamekeepers" Thumb

Clin Sports Med 1998;17:553

Cause: Hyperabduction of the thumb MCP joint (eg, the classical fall on a ski pole causing the thumb to be held while the remainder of the hand plunges into the snow).

Epidem:
- Initially observed in Scottish gamekeepers who would kill hares by placing the thumb and index fingers around the neck to hyperextend it.

- The injury is now almost exclusively traumatically induced in sports such as skiing.

Pathophys:
- Ulnar collateral ligament sprain—4 classes:
    - Type 1: avulsion fx, non-displaced
    - Type 2: avulsion fx, displaced
    - Type 3: torn ligament, stable in flexion
    - Type 4: torn ligament, unstable in flexion

Sx: Pain over the UCL area, weak and painful pinch.

Si:
- Initiated with stress testing.
- Tenderness and swelling over the ulnar aspect of the thumb MCP.
- Stress testing should be performed if there is no evidence of avulsion fracture and is performed as follows:
    - The area is anesthetized with either a local block or median and radial nerve blocks at the wrist.
    - The thumb metacarpal is stabilized with one hand and a valgus stress placed on the MCP with the MCP in full flexion. Testing is done in full flexion because with extension or slight flexion the normally taut volar plate gives the MCP stability.
    - Complete rupture (type 4) is suspected if there is angulation 15° > than the normal thumb or an absolute angulation of >35°.
    - Angulation less than described above is type 3 and considered stable.

X-ray:
- Radiographs performed prior to any stress testing in order to reveal any avulsion fragment. If avulsion fracture evident, stress testing should not be done. Displaced fracture >2 mm or rotated fracture should be considered type 4.

- Arthrogram will show extravasation of dye in complete ruptures.

Rx:

- Initially treated with PRICEMM and analgesics, as needed.
- Type 1: thumb spica cast with MCP in full extension for 4 w.
- Type 2: refer for ORIF.
- Type 3: thumb spica cast with IP free and MCP flexed 20° for 3 w.
- Type 4: refer for ORIF.

Fractures

7.9   Middle Phalangeal Fracture

Clin Sports Med 1998;17:491

Cause: Direct trauma to finger.

Epidem: Collision or contact sports.

Pathophys:

- Direct trauma or twisting.
- The fractures tend to be transverse, generally angulated palmarly, and are often unstable due to the opposing forces of the dorsal extensor tendon and the FDA palmarly.

Sx: Pain and swelling.

Si:

- Tenderness and swelling over middle phalanx with varying degrees of deformity.
- Always check for rotational deformity.

X-ray: Radiographs show degree of angulation or displacement.

Rx:

- Initially treated with PRICEMM and analgesics, as needed.
- Stable, non-displaced, and non-angulated: buddy tape; use thermoplastic splint for sport activity.
- Stable, minimal angulation: immobilize with the MCP flexed 70°, PIP flexed 45°, DIP free and buddy taping to control rotation. Splint is removed in 3-4 w and ROM exercises begun. The splint is worn during sporting activities for an additional 9-10 w.
- Unstable (displaced, angulated, unable to hold reduction): refer to orthopedics.

7.10 PIP Fracture Dislocation

Clin Sports Med 1998;17:491

Cause: Caused by an axial load on a semi-flexed finger.

Epidem: Collision or contact sports.

Pathophys: The middle phalanx shears dorsally, affecting the palmar articular surface of the middle phalanx with the condyles of the proximal phalanx.

Sx: Pain and swelling over the PIP.

Si: Subtle dorsal prominence over the PIP, with localized tenderness.

X-ray: Radiographs demonstrate the proximal aspect of the middle phalanx to be dorsally displaced and the palmar articular fragment to be maintained palmarly.

Rx:

- Initially treated with PRICEMM and analgesics, as needed.
- Small fragment without dislocation: buddy tape.

- Larger fragment but <40% of articular surface: closed reduction followed by extension block splint with PIP in 30-60° of flexion for 3 w.
- Fragment >40% of articular surface: surgical consultation for ORIF.

7.11 Proximal Phalangeal Fractures

Clin Sports Med 1998;17:491

Cause: Direct trauma.

Epidem: Collision or contact sports.

Pathophys:
- Most fractures are spiral or oblique, tend to shorten, and are therefore unstable.
- These are difficult to treat due to the compact anatomy of extensor hood, lateral bands, and flexor tendons surrounding it.
- Scarring or displacement disturbs the tendon balance.

Sx: Pain, swelling, variable degree of deformity.

Si: Tenderness, swelling, varying degrees of shortening, angulation, or rotation.

X-ray: Radiographs will reveal type and extent of the injury.

Rx:
- Initially treated with PRICEMM and analgesics as needed.
- Fracture stability and early ROM are critical to successful treatment.
- Stable fractures: immobilize with wrist in slight extension, MCP in 70° flexion, PIP and DIP joints free, buddy taping to adjacent finger for 3-4 w. Buddy taping is then continued until asymptomatic.
- Unstable (usual type): refer to orthopedics.

7.12 Metacarpal Fractures

Clin Sports Med 1998;17:491

Cause: Direct trauma from either an axial load or compressive forces.

Epidem: Fifth MC neck fractures common in martial arts, but can occur in any contact or collision sport.

Pathophys:
- Neck fractures tend to angulate volarly to a significant degree. Shaft fractures are frequently stabilized by the intrinsic muscles.
- 60% are angulated >40° and angulation up to 70° does not result in significant functional disability.
- The 2nd and 3rd digits are necessary for power grip and much less angulation (<10°) is acceptable here than the 4th and 5th.

Sx: Pain and swelling.

Si: Varying degrees of angular or rotational deformity.

X-ray: Radiographs confirm fracture and degree of angulation/displacement.

Rx:
- Initially treated with PRICEMM and analgesics, as needed.
- Reduction technique:
  - Fracture site is anesthetized with hematoma block.
  - The MCP is flexed 90° and the direction and force of the displacement/angulation is reversed.
  - After reduction the wrist is placed in a well-molded ulnar gutter splint incorporating the 4th and 5th fingers with the MCP flexed 70°.
  - Postreduction radiographs should confirm adequate reduction.

- Splint is worn for 4 w and early ROM exercises begun to prevent stiffness.
- Fifth MC neck fractures should be reduced to <40°, esp in boxers or baseball players who may have significant functional compromise with an angulation of 40°.
- Second and 3rd MC neck fractures: should be reduced if angulated >10° and casted with the MCP at 70° for 4 w.
- MC shaft fractures: immobilized with the adjacent finger with the MCP flexed 70° and PIP slightly flexed. Splint is removed after 10 d and active ROM exercises begun. The splint is reapplied if the fracture site remains tender.
- Unstable fractures should be referred to orthopedic surgeon.

7.13 CMC Fracture Dislocation—"Bennett's Fracture"

Clin Sports Med 1998;17:491

Cause: Axial and abduction forces to the thumb.

Epidem: Collision or contact sports.

Pathophys: The anterior oblique CMC ligament holds the palmar fragment in its normal anatomic position. The abductor pollicus longus pulls the MC shaft fragment radial and dorsal.

Sx: Pain and swelling over base of thumb CMC.

Si: Variable degree of deformity over the thumb CMC.

X-ray: PA, lateral, and oblique radiographs will show the palmar fragment ranging in size from a small avulsion fracture to a large triangular fragment.

Rx:
- Initially treated with PRICEMM and analgesics, as needed.
- These are unstable—refer to orthopedics.

Dislocations

7.14 DIP Joint Dislocation

Clin Sports Med 1986;5:757

Cause: Hyperextension, varus or valgus forces.

Epidem: Collision or contact sports.

Pathophys:
- Rare injury due to the short lever arm of the distal phalanx and strong collateral ligaments.
- Often are compound dislocations due to the dense cutaneous ligaments that anchor the overlying skin.

Sx: Pain and swelling over the DIPJ.

Si: Dorsal or lateral angulation of the DIPJ.

X-ray: Radiographs will show the angulation and associated fractures.

Rx:
- Initially treated with PRICEMM, splinting, and analgesics as needed.
- Reduction technique: anesthetize with digital block. Middle phalanx is stabilized with one hand and the dorsal base of the distal phalanx is "pushed" into reduction.
- Postreduction should be splinted in slight flexion for 10-12 d.
- The rare irreducible dislocation should be referred for open reduction.

7.15 PIP Dorsal Dislocation

Clin Sports Med 1986;5:757

Cause: Hyperextension injury with resultant disruption of the volar plate at its attachment to the middle phalanx.

Epidem: Collision or contact sports.

Pathophys: Loss of the volar stabilizing force causes the phalanx to ride dorsally on the proximal phalanx producing a "bayonet" deformity.

Sx: Pain and swelling over PIP.

Si: Deformity and inability to move PIP.

X-ray: Radiographs will reveal a dorsally displaced middle phalanx, parallel to proximal phalanx with some retraction.

Rx:
- Initially treated with PRICEMM, splinting, and analgesics as needed.
- Reduction technique: anesthetize with metacarpal block. Middle phalanx is grasped with one hand, giving slight hyperextension of the PIP. The other hand grasps the proximal phalanx and that thumb pushes the middle phalanx into reduction. Longitudinal traction of the middle phalanx may allow soft tissue interposition into the PIP and should be avoided.
- Postreduction should be placed in dorsal extension block splint with PIP blocked at 20-30° of flexion but allowed to flex for 3 w. Follow with buddy taping until symptoms resolve.

7.16 PIP Palmar Dislocation

Clin Sports Med 1986;5:757

Cause: Torsional or shearing stress applied to a semi-flexed joint.

Epidem: Collision or contact sports.

Pathophys:
- The above forces result in rupture of one collateral ligament from its proximal attachment and the central slip insertion allowing the proximal phalangeal condyle to buttonhole through the torn extensor mechanism.
- The torn collateral ligament may become entrapped between the middle and proximal phalanges preventing closed reduction.

Sx: Pain and swelling over the PIP.

Si: Tenderness over the PIP, especially dorsally and on the side. Varying degrees of angular or rotational deformity.

X-ray: PA, lateral, and oblique radiographs show volar displacement of the middle phalanx.

Rx:

- Initially treated with PRICEMM, splinting, and analgesics, as needed.
- Closed reduction may be attempted, but these are frequently irreducible or unstable. If reduction is successful (postreduction films show normal congruence of joint surfaces), the treatment is same as for central slip avulsions.
- Irreducible dislocations should be referred to orthopedics.

7.17 MCP Dislocation

Clin Sports Med 1997;16:705

Cause: Torsional or shear forces across the MCP.

Epidem: Collision or contact sports.

Pathophys:

- Simple dislocations: the volar plate remains attached and the proximal phalanx rests perpendicular to the MC.
- Complex dislocation: the MC head goes through the volar plate causing a buttonhole effect, and rests between the lumbricals radially and long flexors ulnarly.

Sx: Pain, swelling, and stiffness at the MCP joint.

Si:

- Variable degree of deformity.
- Simple dislocations: the proximal phalanx is dorsally angulated 60-90°.

- Complex dislocations are subtler appearing with the involved digit (usually the index finger) slightly hyperextended and ulnar deviated with dimpling on the palmar surface of the MCP.

X-ray:
- Simple dislocation: lateral view shows hyperextended MCP.
- Complex dislocation: PA shows widened joint space with asymmetric inclination of proximal phalanx toward the more ulnar finger. Lateral view may show sesamoid interposition between proximal phalanx and MC.

Rx:
- Initially treated with PRICEMM, splinting, and analgesics as needed.
- Simple dislocation: same technique as for PIP dorsal dislocation.
- Complex dislocation: reduction may be attempted if injury is acute and no swelling has occurred.
  - The deformity is exaggerated and the base of the proximal phalanx is pushed over the articular surface. No longitudinal traction is applied as this will tighten the entrapment described under anatomy. Once reduced, this is stable and the finger is buddy taped and early ROM begun.
  - These are generally irreducible and should be referred to orthopedics.

Lacerations

7.18 Extensor Tendon Laceration

Cause: Laceration over the extensor tendon.

Epidem: Hockey, field hockey, lacrosse, collision or contact sports.

Pathophys: Extension is still possible via the lumbricals and extensor juncturae tendinum if the MCP is flexed.

Sx: Bleeding, pain, inability to straighten finger.

Si:
- Laceration over tendon, tendon edges may be visualized.
- Inability to actively extend the PIP and DIP joints with the MCP in full extension.
- Passive ROM is full.

X-ray: Radiographs may show an associated fracture.

Rx:
- Debride and irrigate wound.
- Wrist is splinted in extension with a volar splint to relax the tendon and referral is made within 48 hr.

7.19 Flexor Tendon Laceration

Cause: Laceration over flexor tendon.

Epidem: Hockey, field hockey, lacrosse, collision or contact sports.

Pathophys:
- Flexor tendons course through an intricate system of pulleys and sheaths.
- Neurovascular bundle is in close proximity.

Sx: Bleeding, pain, inability to flex finger.

Si:
- Laceration over flexor tendon.
- Inability to actively flex DIP (profundus) or PIP (superficialis).
- Capillary refill may be delayed with vascular injury.
- Two-point discrimination will be abnormal with nerve injury.

X-ray: Radiographs may show an associated fracture.

Rx:
- Thorough irrigation and debridement of wound.
- Skin may be closed loosely with interrupted 5-0 nylon and the wrist splinted dorsally in 45° flexion with the MCPs 60-80° and IPs slightly flexed.

- Patients should be referred to a hand surgeon no later than 48 hr.

7.20 Fingertip or Nail Laceration

Cause: Result from direct trauma.

Epidem: Collision or contact sports.

Pathophys: Lacerations may involve the nail, nail bed, small avulsions of the pulp, larger pulp amputations, or bony amputations.

Sx: Bleeding, pain.

Si: Laceration, avulsion, or amputation.

X-ray: Radiographs will document bone involvement.

Rx:
- Initially treat with protective dressing and analgesics as needed.
- Document tetanus status. Dirty wounds may warrant coverage with a first-generation cephalosporin.
- Laceration: irrigate and debride under digital nerve block. Close with simple interrupted 5-0 nonabsorbable.
- Small amputations (<1): thorough irrigation and sterile dressing.
- Larger amputations: irrigate, sterile dressing, and refer immediately to hand surgeon.
- Bony amputation: place amputated part in waterproof bag, then in ice water. Do not soak directly in ice water. Refer to orthopedics.
- Lacerated nails: trim or remove nail. If nail bed is involved, it must be repaired. The nail is removed and the nail bed repaired using 5-0 or 6-0 absorbable sutures.

Infections

7.21 Flexor Tenosynovitis

Cause: Puncture wound or laceration over flexor mechanism.

Epidem: Rock climbing, mountaineering, collision or contact sports.

Pathophys: Flexor sheath provides a tight lubricated path for the tendon to glide. When infected, the sheath fills with pus and rapidly progresses to a deep palmar space infection.

Sx: Pain with finger flexion, swelling.

Si: Overlying puncture wound or laceration, tenderness over flexor tendon sheath, symmetric swelling of the digit, pain with passive extension, flexed position of the digit.

X-ray: Radiographs may show soft tissue swelling.

Rx: Immediate referral for incision and irrigation.

7.22 Septic Arthritis

Cause: Penetrating trauma.

Epidem: Rock climbing, mountaineering, collision or contact sports.

Pathophys:
- Open skin wound either with or without communication with a joint (septic arthritis or cellulitis, respectively).
- Most commonly secondary to "clenched fist" lacerations over 4th or 5th MCP joints. Organisms: *Eikenella corrodens*, anaerobes, *Staphylococci*, and *Streptococci* for human bites. *Pasteurella multicida* for animal bites.
- Skin laceration communicates with the joint space allowing for infection.

Sx: Swelling and pain over involved joint.

Si: Tenderness and erythema over involved joint. Pain with axial compression with septic joint.

X-ray: Radiographs may show associated fracture or possibly air in joint.

Lab: CBC, ESR, and cultures. Methylene blue dye can be injected into the joint to look for extravasation, if capsular disruption is suspected.

Rx:

- Septic arthritis: refer immediately to orthopedics.
- Cellulitis: penicillin plus first-generation cephalosporin or ampicillin/clavulanic acid.

7.23 Palmar Space Infection

Cause: Laceration or puncture wound to palmar area.

Epidem: Rock climbing, mountaineering, collision or contact sports.

Pathophys: Can involve the web space, deep space of the thenar space, midpalmar space or Parona's space in the wrist.

Sx: Pain, redness, warmth over involved area.

Si: Associated puncture wound or laceration, tenderness.

X-ray: Radiographs usually normal, may show embedded foreign body.

Lab: CBC, ESR. Cultures should be obtained prior to antibiotic therapy.

Rx:

- Tetanus toxoid, as needed.
- Surgical drainage.
- Culture directed postoperative antibiotics.

Chapter 8

Wrist Injuries

Fractures and Osseous Injury

8.1 Scaphoid Fracture

AAOS Instr Course Lect 2003;52:197; Clin Sports Med 1998;17:469

Cause: Falling on an outstretched hand resulting in hyperextension of wrist.

Epidem:
- Most common carpal fracture.
- Accounts for more than 70% of carpal fractures.

Pathophys:
- Scaphoid bridges proximal and distal carpal rows and serves key stabilizing role in wrist.
- Unique blood supply feeding from distal end results in slower healing in mid- and proximal fractures.
- Three main types: distal or tuberosity, waist, proximal pole.

Sx:
- Pain in anatomic snuffbox after appropriate mechanism.
- Pain with extension of wrist and firm grip.

Si:
- Swelling and occasionally bruising is seen.
- Marked tenderness to palpation in anatomic snuffbox.
- Pain with extremes of extension, flexion, and ulnar deviation.

Diff Dx:

- de Quervain's tenosynovitis (see 8.6); carpal or carpal-metacarpal DJD; instabilities (see 8.10).

Crs: Frequent delayed union or nonunion.

X-ray:

- Initial x-ray often negative. Repeat image in 2 w may demonstrate fracture.
- Three-phase bone scan will demonstrate occult fracture 72 hr after injury.
- MRI can demonstrate fracture earlier.

Rx:

Initial treatment is PRICEMM and thumb spica splint:

- **P**rotection, bracing or splinting
- **R**est, relative rest from offending activities
- **I**ce, for pain management and to reduce swelling
- **C**ompression, to reduce swelling
- **E**levation, to control swelling
- **M**edications, NSAIDs and/or narcotics
- **M**odalities, through physical therapy for pain management and to control swelling.

In nondisplaced fracture, thumb spica cast for 6-12 w, until clinical healing is demonstrated, is the rule. Sources differ regarding long arm or short arm casting. Most typically, long arm for 4 w, followed by short arm until healed.

Displaced fractures, proximal fractures, and nonunions required surgical pinning.

8.2 Hamate Fracture

Clin Sports Med 1998;17:469

Cause: Direct blow to hypothenar eminence fractures hook.

Epidem: Relatively rare, but occurs in baseball, club and racquet sports, and martial arts.

Pathophys:
- Most commonly fractured at the hook, which may lead to ulnar nerve injury.
- Fracture of the body can occur in conjunction with dorsal metacarpal dislocation.

Sx:
- Pain, swelling, and bruising at hypothenar eminence.
- May have numbness along 5th digit (deep branch of ulnar nerve).

Si: Tenderness at hamate/hook.

X-ray:
- Radiographs usually diagnostic. Carpal tunnel view for hook fractures, oblique wrist films for body.
- CT or tomograms may be useful if not visualized on plain radiographs.

Rx:
- Hook fractures often require surgical extraction of hook.
- Nondisplaced body fractures treated with short arm cast for 4-6 w. Displaced fractures require wire fixation.

Return to Activity:
- Usually can play with appropriate cast as symptoms allow.
- Bracing and physical therapy following casting.

8.3   Triquetrum Fracture (Chip Fracture)

Hand Clin 1988;4:469; AAOS Instr Course Lect 1985;34:314

Cause: Hyperextension injury with impaction on the ulnar styloid (fall on outstretched hand) or direct blow to dorsal hand.

Epidem: Roller sports, contact sports, martial arts.

Pathophys: Impingement on ulnar styloid frequently causes dorsal chip fracture.

Sx: Dorsal wrist pain, swelling, bruising is common.

Si:
- Tender at dorsal hand over triquetrum.
- Pain with active extension or passive flexion.

Crs:
- Symptoms typically resolve with short arm casting.
- Nonunion of chip fracture is relatively common but seldom symptomatic.

X-ray: Avulsion usually visualized on true lateral or oblique film.

Rx:
- Short arm cast for 3-4 w usually adequate.
- Persistent symptoms may require excision of fragment.

Return to Activity:
- Usually can play with appropriate cast as symptoms allow.
- Bracing and physical therapy following casting.

8.4 Lunate Osteonecrosis (Keinböch's Disease)

Ortho Clin North Am 1986;17:461

Cause: Unknown.

Epidem:
- Associated with repetitive compressive forces (gymnastics, cheerleading).
- Typically in younger athletes.

Pathophys:
- Micro stress fractures with subsequent loss of blood supply leads to AVN.
- Associated with ulnar minus wrist, which increases compressive forces on lunate.
- Stahl classifications:
  Stage 1: acute (normal x-ray, MRI positive)
  Stage 2: sclerotic changes
  Stage 3: lunate collapse
  Stage 4: pancarpal arthrosis/instability

Sx:
- Initially present with vague aching pain, which increases in severity.
- Complain of stiffness.
- Usually no history of substantial trauma.

Si:
- Tenderness at lunate.
- Nonspecific painful range of motion.

Crs: Can continue to progress to complete collapse of lunate with severe arthrosis and carpal instability.

X-ray:
- Initial films are normal or may show nonspecific sclerosis or degenerative cysts. Eventually show progressing sclerosis and collapse of the lunate.
- MRI is study of choice for early diagnosis.

Rx:
- Should be immobilized and referred to a hand specialist for evaluation.
  - Stage 1: Lunate decompression through radial shortening or ulnar lengthening procedures. Revascularization procedures are also advocated.
  - Stage 2, 3: Silicone implant and scapho-trapezial-trapezoid arthrodesis.
  - Stage 4: Proximal row carpectomy.

8.5 Distal Radius Fracture

Clin Sports Med 1998;17:469

Cause:
- Falling on an outstretched hand most common.
- Also direct trauma or forced wrist extension.

Epidem:
- Account for >15% of fractures seen in the emergency room.
- Common in snowboarders, skating, roller sports, and collision sports.

Pathophys:
- Extra-articular fractures from relatively low energy trauma generally results in fracture to metaphysis (Colle's fracture).
- Intra-articular fractures are more common in athletes and arise from high-energy axial load. Results in 4-part comminution in predictable pattern involving:
  - Radial shaft
  - Radial styloid
  - Dorsal medial fragment
  - Palmar medial fragment
- The majority of these comminuted intra-articular fractures are unstable and will require specialty consultation.

Sx:
- Pain, swelling, bruising, deformity at radial wrist.
- Numbness, tingling, or dysesthesias may occur.

Si:
- Tenderness about the distal radius, swelling, bruising, deformity at radial wrist.
- Neurologic and vascular exam may demonstrate compromise.

Crs:
- Stable fractures heal in 4-6 w with cast immobilization.
- Unstable fractures usually require surgical fixation.

X-ray:
- Assess degree of angulation and displacement of metaphyseal fractures.
- AP, lat, oblique generally sufficient to demonstrate intra-articular fractures.

- Tomograms are useful to evaluate die-punch lesions of articular radius.

Rx:

- Stable metaphyseal fractures without angulation can be managed with cast immobilization for 6 w. Some prefer a long arm for initial 2-3 w. Serial radiographs should be obtained weekly for the first 3 w to ensure no change in alignment.
- Angulated metaphyseal fractures tend to be unstable after reduction. These can be treated with a well-molded long arm cast for 4 w followed by short arm for an additional 2 w. These fractures must be followed closely for loss of reduction. Surgical fixation is usual preferred method of treatment.
- Intra-articular fractures are usually unstable and should be seen by an orthopedic surgeon for treatment.

Return to Activity:
- Usually can play with appropriate cast as symptoms allow.
- Bracing and physical therapy following casting.

Tendon Injuries

8.6 de Quervain's Tenosynovitis

Clin Sports Med 1992;11:77

Cause: Repetitive wrist motion.

Epidem: Most common in racquet and throwing sports.

Pathophys:
- Tenosynovitis of the extensor pollicis brevis or abductor pollicis longus.
- Both tendons occupy the 1st dorsal wrist compartment and are generally both involved.

Sx:
- Pain and swelling along the radial wrist.
- Pain with gripping and rotational motions (removing the lid from a jar).

Si:
- Tenderness along extensor thumb, radial wrist, and forearm.
- Pain with resisted thumb abduction or extension.
- Finklestein's test: Thumb is passively flexed beneath the flexed fingers and wrist is passively flexed to the ulnar side. A positive test produces pain in the 1st dorsal wrist compartment (Figure 8.1).

Diff Dx: Scaphoid fracture (see 8.1), carpal or carpal-metacarpal DJD, instabilities.

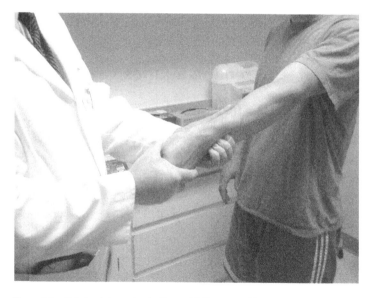

Figure 8.1 Finkelstein's test for de Quervain's Tenosynovitis

Crs:

- Can be insidious onset or acute onset associated with specific event. Chronic pain is common, if untreated.

X-ray:

- Plain radiographs normal.
- MRI may be useful to rule out tendon rupture.

Rx:

- PRICEMM (see 8.1) for pain relief.
- Protective bracing with a thumb spica splint.
- Physical therapy to address strength and flexibility issues.
- Corticosteroid injection (see 1.3).
- Surgical treatment involving a synovectomy may be necessary in persistent cases.

Return to Play:

- With protective splinting as symptoms allow.

8.7 Intersection Syndrome

Clin Sports Med 1992;11:77

Cause: Usually from overuse.

Epidem: Most common in racquet or throwing sports, but can occur with direct trauma in any activity.

Pathophys: Intersection comprised of extensor pollicis brevis, abductor pollicis longus, and the wrist extensors.

Sx: Pain along dorsoradial wrist. Worse with gripping, or twisting motion in wrist.

Si:

- Tenderness and often swelling along dorsoradial forearm at the junction of the distal and middle thirds.
- May have local crepitus with wrist extension.

- Pain localized to this area with resisted extension of wrist or abduction/extension of the thumb.

Crs: Usually insidious onset and chronic symptoms.

X-ray: Plain radiographs normal.

Rx:
- PRICEMM for pain relief (see Rx in Section 8.1).
- Protective bracing with wrist in neutral or slight dorsiflexion.
- Physical therapy to address strength and flexibility issues.
- Corticosteroid injection: After sterile preparation, 1 cc triamcinolone (40 mg/cc) with 1 cc lidocaine is injected into the tendon sheaths at the point of tenderness.
- Surgical treatment rarely indicated.

Return to Play: With protective splinting, as symptoms allow.

8.8   Extensor Carpi Ulnaris (ECU) Tendinitis

Clin Sports Med 1992;11:77

Cause: Injury from acute strain or repetitive motion injury to ECU tendon.

Epidem: Most commonly seen in golf, racquet sports, and wrestling.

Pathophys:
- ECU is contained in the 6th dorsal wrist compartment.
- Arises from acute strain or subluxation resulting from eccentric radial deviation or hypersupination of the wrist respectively, or repetitive motion.
- Often confused with TFCC injury.

Sx:
- May describe an acute strain injury (such as doffing a ball in golf) or a repetitive activity involving wrist radial/ulnar deviation.
- Pain at ulnar wrist exacerbated by wrist extension or ulnar deviation.

Si:
- Tenderness at ulnar wrist may be hard to distinguish from TFCC tear.
- Pain with resisted ulnar deviation and passive radial deviation.
- Pain with resisted wrist extension.

Diff Dx: TFCC tear (see 8.13), ulnar styloid fracture, dorsal impaction syndrome (see 8.14).

X-ray:
- X-rays negative
- MRI may show tenosynovitis and will help distinguish from TFCC tear.

Rx:
- PRICEMM (see 8.1).
- Bracing.
- Corticosteroid injection may be helpful (see 1.4).

Return to Play:
- With protective splinting, as symptoms allow.

8.9   Flexor Tenosynovitis

Clin Sports Med 1998;17:433

Cause: Can arise from single eccentric overload event, more commonly from repetitive overuse.

Epidem: Gripping activities (cycling, racquet sports, batting, and golf).

Pathophys:
- Three distinct tendon groups:
  - Flexor digitorum
  - Flexor carpi ulnaris
  - Flexor carpi radialis
- Inflammation of the tendons may result in compressive neuropathies.

- Flexor digitorum: Carpal tunnel syndrome (see 15.8).
- Flexor carpi ulnaris: Ulnar neuropathy (see 15.10).

Sx:

- Pain localized to flexor compartment(s), which may include length of forearm. Aching pain often at rest following activity.
- Pain with active flexion or passive extension of the wrist.
- Neurologic symptoms (numbness, tingling) with FD or FCU.

Si:

- Tenderness localized to involved tendon.
- Manual muscle testing produces pain localized to specific tendon.
- Neurologic examination may demonstrate compressive neuropathy.

X-ray: Usually normal.

Special Testing:

- EMG useful for CTS (flexor digitorum) and ulnar neuropathy (FCU).

Rx:

- PRICEMM (see 8.1).
- Bracing or casting (recalcitrant symptoms).
- Physical or occupational therapy to improve ROM and strength. Eccentric exercise probably most effective.
- Corticosteroid injection:
  - CTS (flexor digitorum): 1 cc triamcinolone (40 mg /cc) in 1 cc lidocaine into the carpal tunnel (see 1.6).
  - Flexor radialis: 1½ cc triamcinolone (40 mg /cc) in 1½ cc lidocaine into the tendon sheath.
  - Flexor carpi ulnaris: 1½ cc triamcinolone (40 mg /cc) in 1½ cc lidocaine into the tendon sheath.
- Surgery:
  - Carpal tunnel release.
  - Tendon sheath synovectomy for stenosing tenosynovitis.

8.10 Common Extensor Tenosynovitis

Clin Sports Med 1998;17:433

Cause: Overuse, infection from penetrating trauma, rheumatologic conditions, and acute strain injury.

Epidem:
- Less common than other wrist tendinopathies in the athlete.
- More commonly related to vocational duties.

Pathophys: Common extensors reside in the 4th dorsal wrist compartment.

Sx:
- Painful swelling in dorsal midline wrist.
- Pain with motion in the wrist that extends into 4th dorsal compartment of forearm.

Si:
- "Goose foot sign" erythema and swelling on dorsal wrist and hand involving the tendon sheath of the extensor tendons.
- Pain with resisted extension of fingers at the MCP joints.

Lab: Without history of trauma, screening rheumatologic tests indicated including ESR, RF, and ANA.

X-ray: Radiographs negative.

Rx:
- PRICEMM.
- Neutral wrist splint or casting in recalcitrant cases.
- Physical therapy to improve tendon glide and flexibility may be helpful.
- Decompressive surgery for stenosing tenosynovitis may be required.

Return to Play: As symptoms allow.

Ligament Injuries

8.11 Scapholunate Dissociation

Clin Sports Med 1998;17:533

Cause: Fall on an outstretched hand.

Epidem:
- Most common type of carpal instability.
- Collision sports, skiing, snowboarding, gymnastics.

Pathophys:
- Disruption of the scapholunate interosseous ligament.
- Allows nonsynchronous movement of the lunate in relation to scaphoid.

Sx:
- Painful swelling at dorsal wrist.
- Painful motion especially with radial deviation of wrist.

Si:
- Tenderness and swelling at scapholunate articulation.
- Watson shift test: examiner places thumb on distal pole of scaphoid on athlete's palm. As the wrist is moved into a radially deviated position, the normal scaphoid will flex against the examiner's thumb. In SL instability, the examiner can prevent scaphoid flexion. This is painful.

Crs: Chronic instability leads to progressive degeneration within the proximal row most noted at radioscaphoid articulation. Eventually leads to collapse of scaphoid.

X-ray:
- Initial radiographic findings may be subtle with slight increase in scapholunate space (> 3mm). Ring sign: scaphoid is flexed on PA view and will appear short with a ring appearance due to the end-on projection of the cortex.

- Lateral view may demonstrate a dorsal intercalated segment instability (DISI) with the lunate dorsally angulated in relation to the scaphoid.
- MRI arthrogram of the wrist may be useful to delineate anatomy of the injury.

Rx:
- Initial treatment with protective splinting, ice, and pain management.
- Should be evaluated by a hand surgeon relatively early following injury.

8.12 Triquetro-Lunate Instability

Clin Sports Med 1998;17:567

Cause: Typically from a fall on an outstretched hand.

Epidem:
- Less common than scapholunate injuries.
- Collision sports, skiing, snowboarding, cycling, motor sports, martial arts.

Pathophys:
- Three major stabilizers: LT interosseous ligament, volar radiolunotriquetral ligament, and dorsal radiocarpal ligament.
- Injuries range from sprain (no tear of ligament), partial tear, to complete disruption.
- Major instability requires disruption of at least 2 stabilizers; can lead to VISI (volar intercalated segment instability).
- Lesser injuries will cause pain and late stage DJD, but may not be apparent acutely.

Sx:
- Pain at dorsoulnar aspect of wrist.
- Pain with flexion or extension.

Si:

- Tenderness at triquetrolunate articulation.
- Lunotriquetral ballotment test: Examiner stabilizes the lunate with one hand while exerting a volar-dorsal stress on the triquetrum with the other. Pain or instability suggest a positive test.

Crs: In occult injuries (without frank VISI deformity) diagnosis may be delayed. These cases result in chronic pain and degenerative joint disease.

X-ray:

- Plain radiographs may demonstrate instability (VISI) with major injury. Usually normal.
- Wrist MRI arthrography can demonstrate even partial disruption of the supporting ligaments.

Rx:

- Minor injuries without instability may be treated with immobilization for 3-4 w followed by bracing for activity.
- In the subacute setting, corticosteroid injection may be helpful for pain management. 1½ cc triamcinolone (40 mg/cc) in 2 cc anesthetic are injected into the intra-articular space under sterile technique.
- With severe instability or with chronic pain, wrist arthroscopy should be considered.

Other Problems

8.13 TFCC Tear

Clin Sports Med 1998;17:567

Cause:

- Fall on an outstretched hand.
- Hyperrotation of wrist or forearm.

Epidem:

- Degenerative injuries relatively common in gymnasts with ulna plus wrists.
- Acute tears with wrist hyperextension (roller sports, collision sports).
- Avulsion injuries with forced wrist rotation (wrestling, golf, racquet sports).

Pathophys:

- Degenerative disease from repetitive overload to central TFCC (thinnest portion of complex) due to impaction of triquetrum on ulna.
- Acute tear frequently due to compressive forces between the lunate and the ulna in hyperextension injury.
- Avulsion of TFCC from ulna (may include ulnar styloid) results from hyperrotational injury.

Sx:

- Ulnar-sided pain following appropriate mechanism of injury.
- Swelling and bruising may be seen.
- Pain with gripping or manipulation.

Si:

- Tenderness at carpi-ulnar interspace.
- Pain precipitated with passive pronation, supination, and ulnar deviation. Palpable click may accompany pain.
- Assess stability of distal radial ulnar joint (DRUJ).
  - Shuck test: examiner grasps radius in one hand and distal ulna in the other. Volar directed force is applied to the distal radius and degree of motion is compared to the contra-lateral side.

Crs: Frequently results in chronic relapsing ulnar wrist pain.

X-ray:

- Plain radiographs useful to assess ulnar variance and for presence of distal ulna fracture.
- MRI arthrogram can demonstrate tear.

Rx:

- TFCC tear with DRUJ instability should be managed surgically.
- TFCC tear without instability: Initially treated with cast or brace immobilization in slight ulnar deviation/flexion for 4 w. Followed by wrist ROM and strengthening with protective bracing for activities.
- Typically seen in the chronic phase without previous diagnosis or treatment. Treatment in this case includes 2-4 w immobilization. Corticosteroid injection is useful for analgesia (see 1.5).
- Arthroscopic treatment often required.

8.14 Dorsal Impaction Syndrome

Clin Sports Med 1998;17:611

Cause: Repetitive loading of wrist with superphysiologic loads.

Epidem: Gymnasts, cheerleaders.

Pathophys:

- Loaded hyperextension leads to chronic synovitis (meniscoid of the wrist) or microscopic injury to osteocartilage.
- Typically involves scaphoid or lunate, which may develop proximal dorsal ridge.

Sx: Pain with wrist extension.

Si:

- Tenderness at proximal middorsal wrist.
- Pain in this area with wrist extension.

X-ray: Usually normal, but may demonstrate hypertrophic bone of the proximal scaphoid, lunate or at distal radius.

Rx:

- Initial treatment involves limitation of hyperextension. A functional brace (eg, "Lions Paw") most often successful.

- Corticosteroid injection at the site of injury also often helpful; 1 cc (40 mg/cc) triamcinolone in 1 cc lidocaine.
- Persistent cases may respond to cast immobilization with activity avoidance for 3-6 w.
- Surgery may be indicated to debride ossicle in chronic cases.

8.15 Wrist Ganglion

Cause: Frequently idiopathic, may arise after trauma (either acute or repetitive).

Epidem:
- Most common tumor of the wrist. Usually seen on dorsal wrist (scapholunate joint).
- More common in sports with repetitive wrist loading (gymnastics, cheerleading), but seen in athletes of all sports.

Pathophys:
- Cyst is continuous with joint capsule and is filled with synovial fluid.
- Occult ganglia tend to be smaller and more painful. Frequently are the causes of vague wrist pain.
- Scapholunate joint most common, but can arise from any joint.

Sx:
- Vague wrist pain may precede appearance of ganglion.
- Complain of mildly tender mass that may be reducible.

Si:
- Mobile mass usually palpable. May be tender.
- Typically transilluminate.
- Pulsatile mass suggestive of aneurysm and should be further evaluated.

Crs: May reduce and recur. Intermittently tender/painful.

X-ray:
- Usually normal.
- MRI may be helpful to evaluate for occult ganglion.

Rx:
- Aspiration may be attempted, but seldom curative.
- Surgical treatment for symptomatic ganglia or for cosmesis or pain management.

Chapter 9

Back Problems

9.1 Mechanical Low Back Pain (LBP)

Adv Stud Med 2004;4:135; Prim Care 2004;31:33; Phy Sportsmed 2001;29:38; Nejm 2001;344:363; Jama 1992;268:760; AHCPR Pub No 95-0642 Dec 1994

Cause: Repetitive overuse or single-event injury (MVA, golf swing, fall).

Epidem:
- Yearly prevalence of 50% with 15-20% presenting for care.
- 60-90% lifetime incidence.
- Most common cause of disability in <45 y/o age group.
- 90% recover in 6-12 w.
- Estimated annual cost of $38-50b.
- 97% are mechanical in origin.

Pathophys:

Anatomy:
- Bony: 3-joint complex at each level (2 facet joints and disc interposed between 2 vertebrae); degeneration of the disc transfers weight-bearing and rotational load to the facet joints causing joint inflammation and degeneration.
- Muscular Anatomy:
  - Anterior group-abdominal and psoas muscles.
  - Posterior group-erector spinae, profundi, and intersegmental muscles.
- ROM: Forward flexion: 90°, extension: 30°, side flexion: 30°, trunk rotation: 70°; these are combined numbers, but most

notable is a reversal of normal lumbar lordosis with forward
bend resulting in a smooth kyphotic bowing of the lower back.
- Most pain generators in the disc, facet joint capsule, anterior
  and posterior longitudinal ligaments, muscles and other supporting ligaments.

Sx:

- Traumatic injury: fall, MVA, lifting or twisting, repetitive
  bending.
- Mild/mod/severe lumbar pain with minimal radiation.
- H/o prolonged sitting with work or travel.
- No "red flags."
  - Fracture: h/o trauma.
  - Infection or cancer: age > 60, weight loss, fever, night pain,
    h/o cancer (bone mets common in breast, lung, thyroid,
    renal, prostate), infection risk factors of iv drug use, immune
    suppression, recent bacterial infection.
- Cauda equina syndrome: saddle anesthesia, bowel or bladder
  dysfunction, progressive neurologic deficit.

Si: Paraspinal muscle tenderness, no bony tenderness, and pain in
back with passive knee-to-chest stretch, limited ability to forward
bend; negative discogenic exam (see 9.2).

Crs: Ninety percent of episodes of mechanical LBP will resolve in 12 w.

Cmplc: Prolonged disability for work, recurrent LBP, inability to participate in sport/recreational activity.

Diff Dx: Discogenic back pain (see 9.2), infection, metastatic disease
(breast, lung, thyroid, renal cell, prostate), cauda equina syndrome,
fracture (acute: spinous process, compression fx; chronic/subacute:
stress fx of pars), SI dysfunction (see 9.3); non-back pain (AAA,
pyelonephritis, posterior penetrating ulcer, pancreatitis).

Lab: If indicated, consider CBC, ESR, and UA.

X-ray:

- Image, if h/o trauma, "red flags," symptoms >1 month.
- Lumbar spine series (AP, LAT, and cone down lateral of L5-S1).

- Bone scan for occult injury or infection.
- MRI usually not necessary.

Rx: See 22.3 for back rehabilitation exercises.

Initial phase:
- Bed rest <48 hr maximum if any.
- Ice massage (15 min every 2 hr) followed by passive knee-to-chest stretch (one leg at a time then both legs together).
- NSAID of choice for 5-7 d.
- Short-term use of narcotic pain meds for severe pain.
- Valium 5 mg tid for 1-2 d for severe spasm.
- Daily walks followed by stretching
- Physical therapy for modalities and stretching.
  - Ice massage.
  - Electrical stimulation.
  - Iontophoresis/phonophoresis.

Second phase:
- Continued pain management.
- Consider low dose TCA (Elavil 10-50 mg hs or Pamelor 10-50 mg hs) for chronic pain (>12 w) and sleep disturbance.
- Survey for "red flags."
- Stretching of hamstrings and back (knee-chest).
- Strengthening of back flexors (abs) and extensors.
- Injection of trigger points (1 cc of 1% lidocaine at each site).

Prevention:
- Aerobic exercise, general conditioning, weight management.
- Proper lifting techniques and posture.
- Core strengthening.

Referral:
- "Red flags" to appropriate consultant asap.
- Physical therapy for rehab and lumbar stabilization program.
- Pain clinic for chronic pain management.
- Chiropractic for manipulative management.
- Osteopath for OMT.

BACK PROBLEMS

Return to Activity: Activity is the cornerstone of therapy (Spine 2002;27:1736); when pt can tolerate flexion/extension activities, has a normal neurologic exam and functional performance of gait, lumbopelvic rhythm on FF, and a desire to return to activity whether it be sport or occupation.

9.2   Discogenic Back Pain

Sciatica or Herniated Nucleus Pulposis (HNP)

Adv Stud Med 2004;4:135; Prim Care 2004;31:33; Am Fam Phys 2000;61:1779; The Low Back Pain Handbook. St. Louis: Mosby 1996:71

Cause: Bending/twisting motion causing herniation of the nucleus pulposis through the annulus fibrosis.

Epidem:
- Middle-aged adults 30-40 y/o.
- Represents about 4% of all LBP patients (Adv Stud Med 2004; 4:135).
- 95% at L4-5 and L5-S1.
- 75% resolve spontaneously within 6 m.
- Cumulative risk of 2nd proven disc during next 20 yr is 8%.
- Most commonly involve L4-5 or L5-S1 with involvement of the L4, L5, or S1 nerve roots.

Pathophys:
- Functional anatomy: disc with central soft nucleus pulposis and surrounding "onion skin" layers of the annulus fibrosis.
- Years of abuse and degenerative change allow cracks and tears in the annulus eventually allowing rupture of the nucleus.
  - Microtears of the annulus present as acute back pain with radiation into the buttocks and Valsalva aggravation of pain, but no distal neuro sx or SLR.
- Injury by bending/twisting forces.

- Radicular pain probably less related to mechanical compression, but more chemical irritation of the nerve root.

Sx:

- Past h/o discogenic or mechanical LBP.
- Onset of symptoms with single-event bend or twist activity.
- Pain usually in the buttock or SI area or leg.
- Pain with Valsalva (cough, sneeze, lift, bowel movement).
- Distal neuro complaints of weakness, pain, or paresthesia.
- May or may not have evidence of bowel or bladder symptoms (urinary retention more common).

Si:

- Back usually asymptomatic (if pt has back pain it is probably secondary myofascial pain).
- Pain in sciatic notch (½ way between the greater trochanter and ischium).
- Positive SLR (straight leg raise: pt supine and knee extended, as the leg is elevated between 30 and 70° pain radiating posteriorly below the knee).
- Symptoms aggravated by dorsiflexion of foot.
- Distal neuro findings:

	Motor	**Reflex**	**Sensory**
L3	Hip flexors	patellar	medial thigh
L4	Tibialis anterior quads	patellar	medial leg/foot
L5	Extensor halucus longus (EHL)	none	dorsal foot
S1	Peroneals foot plantarflexion	achilles	lateral foot

N.B.: Test the gastroc-soleus complex by having the patient perform repetitive toe raises and compare to opposite side or may walk in office on heels then toes.

- Spinal reflexes: anal wink, cremasteric, rectal tone.

Crs: Eighty-five percent symptomatic discs resolve in 12 w with con-servative/nonoperative management.

Cmplc: Permanent nerve damage to spinal root with weakness or paresthesia, chronic pain, central disc/cauda equina.

Diff Dx: Discitis, annular tear, compression fracture, spondylosis, mechanical LBP (see 9.1), SI dysfunction (see 9.3), piriformis syndrome or other gluteal muscular pain, ischial bursitis ham-string pain, gluteal abscess, abdominal path (AAA, posterior per-forating ulcer, pancreatitis).

Lab: Usually not necessary.

X-ray: HNP is a clinical diagnosis, radiographs for "red flags" or h/o trauma; MRI should be considered if sx >4-6 w, severe motor loss (foot drop or acute quad tone loss); MRI for refractory cases (>10-12 w) or severe neurologic sx (profound weakness or bowel/bladder dysfunction).

Rx:

Initial:
- Pain control with NSAIDs and judicious use of narcotics.
- Short-term bed rest (<48 hrs).
- Consider short course corticosteroids (hold NSAIDs). Prednisone 2 mg/kg/d for 5-7 d.
- Stool softener.

Phase 2:
- Increase activity as tolerated: start walking program.
- Monitor neuro exam.
- Continue NSAID.
- Back rehab (see 22.3).

Referral:
- Severe motor loss and/or bowel/bladder dysfunction should have urgent MRI and referral to ortho spine or neurosurgery.
- Consider referral to anesthesia pain for ESI for refractory pain with a normal neuro exam.

- Consider early referral to PT for pelvic traction or modalities for management of secondary myofascial pain.

Return to Activity:
- Pain free with good back motion.
- Normal strength or stable strength, if there is evidence of motor loss.
- Beware of lifting techniques and activities that involve repetitive bending or trunk twisting.

9.3 Sacroiliac (SI) Dysfunction

Clin J Sport Med 2003;13:252; Pain Prac 2002;2:17; Am Fam Phys 1992;46:1459

Cause: Acute or chronic injury to sacroiliac joint.

Epidem: Forty percent of chronic back pain; 58% associated with some trauma esp activities requiring single-leg stance (golf, running, skating, gymnastics).

Pathophys:
- Functional anatomy: SI joint is a biconcave joint connecting the hemipelvis to the sacrum.
- The SI joint transmits load from the lower extremities to the spine and it does have movement.
- Injury from inflammation, compression/shear forces, hypermobility.

Sx: May be overuse or repetitive trauma; report of landing on single leg stepping off stair or curb with sudden or delayed ipsilateral SI area pain; pain localized with some radiation into the gluteal area; ± Valsalva symptoms; often cyclic and chronic.

Si: May have localized soft tissue pain in SI area; absent discogenic signs; positive SI provocative tests:
- FABER (Flexion/Abduction/External Rotation), aka Patrick Test, of the hip as in the "figure four" position producing ipsilateral SI pain (Figure 9.1).

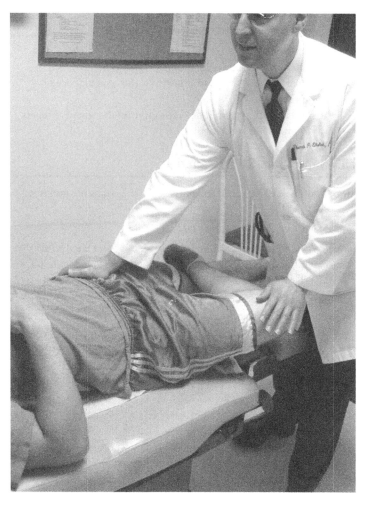

Figure 9.1 FABER Test

- SI compression:
  - Patient on side with affected hip up; downward load applied to the hemipelvis with pain in the affected SI joint.
- Gaenslen's (Figure 9.2):
  - Pt is supine at edge of exam table.
  - The examiner passively flexes one leg to the chest of the pt while the leg near the edge of the table hangs over extending the leg at the hip.
  - Pain in the SI of the hip that is extending is positive.
- Standing extension on single leg (see Figure 16.1):
  - See spondylolysis (see 16.1).
  - The examiner supports the pt as he or she extends a single leg.
  - This is positive with posterior element pain as in spondylolysis, facet arthropathy, spinal stenosis, and SI pain.

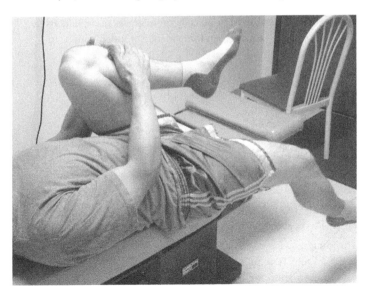

Figure 9.2   Gaenslen's Test

- Gillet's:
  - With the pt standing the examiner places his or her thumb on both PSIS.
  - While the pt elevates each knee to a knee-chest position the examiner assess the degree or absence of normal inferior motion of the PSIS.
  - Decreased motion is an indication of a locked SI joint.

Cmplc: Chronic pain and dysfunction.

Diff Dx: Discogenic pain (see 9.2), inflammatory sacroiliitis (spondylo-arthropathy), gluteal abscess or muscular strain, piriformis syndrome, pelvic path (UTI, prostatitis, uterine/ovarian pain radiation, perirectal abscess).

Lab: Consider labs to r/o inflammatory process: CBC with Diff, ESR/CRP, ANA, RF, UA; questionable value of HLA-B27 as screening test.

X-ray: SI views for signs of displacement, sclerosis, or degenerative change; MRI or bone scan for evidence of inflammation in chronic symptoms.

Rx:

Initial phase: Similar to mechanical LBP:
- Ice
- Knee-chest stretch
- NSAIDs
- As needed short-term narcotics
- Soft tissue injections

Second phase:
- SI self-mobilization
- Physical therapy for modalities and manipulation

Chronic:
- SI injection under floroscopy
- OMT/chiropractic manipulation
- Self-mobilization

Referral:
- PT for modalities
- Pain clinic for SI injection and other pain modalities
- OMT/chiropractic
- Rheumatology for evidence of inflammatory arthritis

Return to Activity: Negative or normal provocative tests; tolerance to trial of activity (walking, running, lifting).

9.4 Lumbar Spinal Stenosis

Dis Mon 2005;51:6; Am Fam Phys 2004;70:517; Phy Sportsmed 2003;31:25; Fed Pract 2003;22:83; Am Fam Phys 1998 57:1825; Rheum Disease Clin N Amer 1994;20:471; Clin Orthop Relat Res 1992;279:82

Cause: Progressive spondylosis (degenerative arthritis of disc and facet joints) causing compression of spinal cord and nerve roots.

Epidem:
- 1:100 >65 y/o undergo laminectomy annually for this problem.
- 1.7-8% annual prevalence.
- 65-95% reported improvement with surgical management with a 1% complication rate.
- L5 (75%), L4 (15%), L3 (5.3%), and L2 (4%).

Pathophys: Function anatomy: osteophyte formation and synovial hypertrophy, as well as disc narrowing that contribute to narrowing of the spinal canal and neuroforaminae.

Si:
- Arthritis with morning stiffness or stiffness after inactivity.
- Back or lower extremity pain (unilateral or bilateral) with prolonged standing or extension activities (walking downhill, down stairs or looking overhead).
- Relief with sitting for short periods of time; may or may not have bowel or bladder symptoms.
- Rare Valsalva symptoms.

BACK PROBLEMS

- Distal neuro usually normal.
- Pts with back stiffness with standing in one position relieved with motion and no significant limitation of time on their feet when moving are more likely to have lumbar OA (spondylosis) and not spinal stenosis.

Sx: Limited back motion by pain and arthritis (esp in extension); exacerbation of symptoms with extension double leg or single leg; absent SLR; absent SI provocative tests; may have distal neuro findings (see 9.2); look for absence of anal reflex.

Crs: Progression of symptoms is common; degree of impairment and rate of progression is variable.

Cmplc: Irreversible neurologic deficit; chronic pain requiring escalating narcotic pain meds.

Diff Dx: Metastatic disease, discogenic pain (see 9.2), infection, compression fx, spondylosis, retroperitoneal path (PUD, pancreatitis, AAA, pelvic path, pyelonephritis).

Lab: Usually not necessary except to work up the diff dx.

X-ray: Lumbar osteoarthritis on radiograph with evidence of spurring, spondylolisthesis (anterior or posterior), disc narrowing, or neurforaminal narrowing; MRI more definitive imaging study (with or without intrathecal contrast); CT generally not helpful.

Rx:

Acute pain
- Limit standing/extension activities (stair/hill descent).
- Programmed rest stops, if have to be on feet.
- NSAID or COX 2 inhibitor.
- Short course corticosteroid for severe radicular symptoms.

Subacute/chronic
- Epidural steroid injections (ESI).
- Flexion-based rehabilitative exercises and core strengthening (see 22.3).

- Cushioned shoes/insoles
- Low impact aerobics
- Bike, Stairmaster, aqua-aerobics

Referral:
- Anesthesia pain for ESI (usually a series of 3 injections).
- Neurosurgery for refractory pain or bowel/bladder/motor symptoms in pt with good operative risk.

Return to Activity: Long-term management should try to limit high-impact activity and, depending on symptoms, avoid repetitive bending and twisting.

Chapter 10

Hip Pain

Anterior Hip and Groin

10.1 Femoral Stress Fracture

Int J Sports Med 1993;14:347; Skeletal Radiol 1986;15:133; Clin
  Orthop 1994;303:155

Cause: Typically follows change in training volume or intensity.

Epidem: Most common in running sports. Amenorrheic females are
  particularly susceptible.

Pathophys:
  - Imbalance between osteoblastic and osteoclastic cell activity
    with bone reabsorption outpacing bone formation leading to
    weakening of cortex.
  - Femoral neck injuries classified as distractive (superior cortex)
    and compressive (inferior cortex).
  - Related to intrinsic factors (foot mechanics, poor flexibility,
    muscle imbalance, coxa vara, etc) and extrinsic factors (run-
    ning surface, shoe selection, etc).

Sx: Vague, increasing groin or thigh pain, made worse with activity.
  Late finding is pain with active hip flexion and at rest.

Si:
  - Tenderness in the affected groin.
  - Pain with a single-leg stance.
  - Passive internal rotation of the hip is painful.
  - Pain with active hip flexion common late finding.

Crs: Insidious onset with gradual worsening pain. If untreated can result in frank fracture. Return to play time variable.

Diff Dx: Femoral head avascular necrosis (see 10.2), acetabular labral tear (see 10.3), adductor strain/tendinitis (see 10.5), iliopectineal bursitis (see 10.4), iliopsoas tendon strain (see 10.6), osteitis pubis (see 10.7).

X-ray:

- Plain radiographs are usually normal in early stress reaction, may demonstrate cortical sclerosis or frank fracture in later studies.
- Triple-phase bone scan is very sensitive even in early stress fractures.
- MRI is useful in diagnosing stress fractures and may be less expensive than bone scan.

Rx: Based on location of injury.

- Femoral neck-distraction cortex: treat aggressively, refer early. Often requires surgical treatment.
- Femoral neck-compression side: the main treatment is rest, followed with periodic plain radiographs to document healing.
- Crutch ambulation with toe-to-floor weight bearing for 6-12 w is the norm.
- Minimum of 6 w required before the pt can gradually resume normal weight-bearing activity.
- Physical therapy directed at improved flexibility and balanced muscle strengthening should be employed, as symptoms allow.
- Pts should be referred to an orthopedic surgeon if symptoms persist, there is evidence of fracture on plain radiograph, or if there is evidence of avascular necrosis on any study.
- Femoral shaft and pubis stress fracture treatment includes rest and activity substitution using pain as a guide (advise the pt to exercise to pain, not through pain). Rarely requires surgical intervention.

10.2 Femoral Head Avascular Necrosis

Orthopedics 1994;17:789; Semin Arthroplasty 1991;2:241

Cause: Most often not identified.

Epidem: Predisposing factors include: prolonged corticosteroid use, heavy alcohol abuse, stress injury or fracture. Over 50% are idiopathic.

Pathophys: Loss of normal vascular watershed involving all or part of femoral head, resulting in tissue death.

Sx:
- Insidious onset of atraumatic groin and anterior leg pain.
- Present at rest, worse with activity.
- May be bilateral.

Si:
- Tenderness in the affected groin.
- Pain with a single-leg stance.
- Passive internal rotation of the hip is painful.

Crs: Typically progressive pain and development of DJD.

Cmplc: Degenerative joint disease with limited function and chronic pain.

Diff Dx:
- Femoral stress fracture (see 10.1), acetabular labral tear (see 10.3), adductor strain/tendinitis (see 10.5), iliopectineal bursitis (see 10.4), iliopsoas tendon strain (see 10.6), osteitis pubis (see 10.7).

X-ray:
- Plain radiographs normal early, later demonstrate sclerosis, progressive cortical flattening, and degenerative joint disease.
- MRI will demonstrate early disease prior to radiographic changes.

HIP PAIN

Rx:

- Early surgical intervention is possible, including cortical drilling and vascularized bone grafting. Results vary.
- Symptomatic treatment for pain relief.
- Activity modification.
- Total hip arthroplasty for late DJD.

Return to Activity: Minimal weight bearing until symptoms resolve then gradual return to weight-bearing exercise, avoiding pain.

10.3 Acetabular Labral Tear

Orthopedics 1995;18:753; Clin Orthop Relat Res 2003;406:38

Cause: Twisting injury on weight-bearing hip.

Epidem: Incidence unknown. Most common in collision sports.

Pathophys:

- Tear of the fibrocartilaginous ring around peripheral acetabulum.
- Recently described entity thought to be responsible for many cases of chronic anterior hip/groin pain.

Sx:

- Deep, anterior hip pain, intermittently present, typically described as sharp or stabbing.
- May or may not have history of macro-traumatic event.
- Pain is worse with activity.

Si:

- May not have tenderness on palpation.
- Often pain with passive external or internal rotation.
- Thomas flexion-to-extension test: patient lies on the contralateral side with both hips maximally flexed. The affected hip is then moved from full flexion to full extension. Painful click suggests labral tear.

Crs: Frequently chronic anterior hip pain not responsive to treatment. May resolve with decreased activity.

Diff Dx:
- Femoral stress fracture (see 10.1), femoral head avascular necrosis (see 10.2), adductor strain/tendinitis (see 10.5), iliopectineal bursitis (see 10.4), iliopsoas tendon strain (see 10.6), osteitis pubis (see 10.7).

X-ray:
- Plain radiographs normal.
- Diagnostic lidocaine injection (intra-articular) alleviates pain temporarily.
- MRI arthrogram may demonstrate tear.
- Diagnostic arthroscopy is the gold standard.

Rx:
- Trial of PRICEMM (see 1.1) and physical therapy.
- Arthroscopy in cases with persistent pain, although results are variable.

10.4 Iliopectineal Bursitis

J Rheumatol 1995;22:1971

Cause: Overuse injury.

Epidem: Most common in running, dancing, martial arts.

Pathophys:
- Bursa in the deep anterior soft tissues between the iliopectineal eminence and iliopsoas muscle/tendon.
- Inflammation related to overuse, poor flexibility, and abnormal gait mechanics.

Sx:
- Gradual onset of deep anterior hip pain.
- Exacerbated with activity, particularly with hip extension.

Si:
- Tenderness may be reproducible.
- Limp is common.
- Pain with active internal rotation and passive extension of hip.

Crs: Insidious onset, persistent symptoms.

Diff Dx:
- Femoral stress fracture (see 10.1), femoral head avascular necrosis (see 10.2), acetabular labral tear (see 10.3), adductor strain/tendinitis (see 10.5), iliopectineal bursitis (see 10.4), iliopsoas tendon strain (see 10.7), osteitis pubis (see 10.7).

X-ray:
- Plain radiographs usually negative.
- MRI may demonstrate fluid in bursa or inflammatory changes of the iliopsoas tendon.

Rx:
- PRICEMM.
- Physical therapy to address flexibility and gait issues.
- Surgery has been described.

10.5 Adductor Tendon Strain

Sports Med 1998;25:271

Cause: Acute strain injury.

Epidem: Most common in collision or contact sports.

Pathophys: Injury to adductor muscle group caused by eccentric external rotation with hip in abducted position.

Sx:
- Abrupt onset of sharp pain in groin following appropriate injury.
- Continued pain with ambulation, kicking, and jumping.

Si:

- Point tender in groin.
- Pain elicited with passive abduction, active adduction, and resisted internal rotation.

Diff Dx: Femoral stress fracture (see 10.1), femoral head avascular necrosis (see 10.2), acetabular labral tear (see 10.3), iliopectineal bursitis (see 10.4), iliopsoas tendon strain (see 10.6), osteitis pubis (see 10.7).

X-ray: Plain radiographs rule out avulsion injury.

Rx:

- PRICEMM.
- Stretching and strengthening exercise within limits of pain.
- Gradual return to full activities with augmented stretching program for prevention.

10.6 Iliopsoas Tendon Strain

Sports Med 1998;25:271

Cause: Acute strain injury.

Epidem: Common in soccer and football.

Pathophys: Eccentric strain injury caused by forceful contraction of iliopsoas with the foot planted or with hip in extended position.

Sx:

- Abrupt onset of groin pain with appropriate mechanism.
- Pain with active hip flexion (walking or running).

Si:

- Tenderness in affected groin.
- Pain with passive external rotation and active hip flexion.

Crs: Acute onset, fairly debilitating.

Diff Dx: Femoral stress fracture (see 10.1), femoral head avascular necrosis (see 10.2), acetabular labral tear (see 10.3), adductor strain/tendinitis (see 10.5), iliopectineal bursitis (see 10.4), osteitis pubis (see 10.7).

X-ray: Plain radiographs may reveal avulsion fracture from the lesser trochanter in young patients.

Rx:
- Initial PRICEMM.
- Early range of motion within pain-free range.
- Structured therapy for improving strength and flexibility, as symptoms allow.

Return to Activity: Return to play in 1-6 w.

10.7 Osteitis Pubis

Curr Sports Med Rep 2003;2:98; Sports Med 1991;12:266

Cause: Repetitive overload to pelvis (running, jumping, etc).

Epidem:
- Most common in women after childbearing.
- Running, jumping, cutting, and collision sports.

Pathophys:
- Inflammation at the symphysis pubis articulation.
- May be related to early return to sports in postpartum period, or repetitive macrotrauma leading to relative dynamic instability.

Sx: Gradually worsening midline groin pain, worse with activity.

Si:
- Point tender at symphysis pubis.
- Pain in midline with single-leg stance.

Diff Dx:
- Femoral stress fracture (see 10.1), femoral head avascular necrosis (see 10.2), acetabular labral tear (see 10.3), adductor strain/tendinitis (see 10.5), iliopectineal bursitis (see 10.4), iliopsoas tendon strain (see 10.6).

X-ray:
- Plain radiographs may show degenerative changes at synchondrosis.
- Bone scan useful to determine active vs inactive disease at symphysis.

Rx:
- Relative rest until asymptomatic avoiding precipitating activities.
- Nonsteroidal anti-inflammatories.
- Corticosteroid injection: 2 cc triamcinolone (40 mg/cc) in 3 cc topical anesthetic instilled sterilely into articular space.

Return to Activity: When asymptomatic.

Lateral Hip

10.8 Greater Trochanter Bursitis

Mayo Clin Proc 1996;71:565

Cause: Direct trauma or overuse in the setting of SI dysfunction.

Epidem: Common in runners, cross-country skiers and sedentary individuals.

Pathophys:
- Irritation of any of bursa overlying the superior margin of the greater trochanter.
- Usually due to tightness in ITB, arising from poor flexibility, SI dysfunction, leg length discrepancy, or gait anomalies.

- Results from acute trauma, overuse, or mechanical factors, including shortened hip abductors or external rotators, increased varus angulation of the hip due to leg length discrepancy, or a broad pelvic structure.
- Calcific bursitis is occasionally seen.

Sx:

- Deep, aching, lateral hip pain that may extend into the buttocks or down into the lateral knee.
- Pain is aggravated by activity, local pressure or stretching, often worse at night.

Si:

- Palpation over the bony prominence of the greater trochanter, and slightly inferiorly or posteriorly elicits tenderness.
- Pain with resisted hip abduction and external rotation as well.
- Leg length discrepancy common.
- SI tenderness and restricted motion is common.
- Ober's test (Figure 10.1) positive: pt lies on unaffected side, both hips and knees initially flexed, affected hip and knee are extended stressing soft tissues over greater trochanter.

Crs: Frequently chronic or recurrent lateral hip pain.

Diff Dx:

- Trochanteric bursitis (see 10.8), snapping hip syndrome (see 10.9), hip pointer (see 10.10), neuropathies involving the lumbar nerve roots (L2-4) and branches of the iliohypogastric or subcostal nerves, sclerotomal irritation of lumbar facet joints and paraspinal ligaments, and femoral head and neck pathology.

X-ray: Plain radiographs usually normal.

Rx:

- PRICEMM.
- Rehabilitative exercises aimed at improving flexibility of the iliotibial band, SI function, and hip rotator strength.

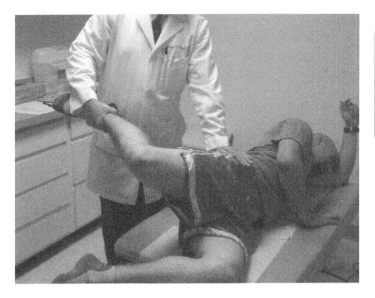

Figure 10.1   Ober Test

- Weight loss, conditioning, and proper lifting technique can aid in preventing recurrent or chronic injury.
- The local injection of corticosteroid is often effective in relieving symptoms. Because of the relatively large volume of this bursa, 10 cc of lidocaine with 80 mg of triamcinolone should be injected at the point of maximal tenderness.

Return to Activity: Should be encouraged and advanced, as symptoms allow.

10.9 Snapping Hip Syndrome

Am J Sports Med 2004;32:1504; J Bone Joint Surg 1991;73:253

Cause: Soft tissue friction over the greater or lesser trochanter.

Epidem:
- Relatively uncommon.
- More frequent in female runners, hurdlers, and gymnasts

Pathophys: Most commonly related to snapping of illiotibial band over greater trochanter (lateral snapping hip) or the iliopsoas tendon snapping over the lesser trochanter.

Sx:
- Painful snapping sensation with hip flexion/extension.
- Groin pain with medial snapping hip syndrome.

Si:
- Prominent palpable or audible snap with hip flexion and extension.
- May reproduce symptoms with flexion, abduction, external rotation (FABER) position (see Figure 9.1).
- Ober's test may be positive (see Figure 10.1).

Crs: Often not painful, but disturbing to athlete. In these cases the response to therapy is variable.

X-ray: Normal.

Rx:
- Physical therapy to improve flexibility and balance rotator strength.
- Correct gait abnormalities.
- Surgery has been described (z-plasty), not commonly done.

Diff Dx: Trochanteric bursitis (see 10.8), snapping hip syndrome (see 10.9), hip pointer (see 10.10), neuropathies involving the lumbar nerve roots (L2-4) and branches of the iliohypogastric or subcostal nerves, sclerotomal irritation of lumbar facet joints and paraspinal ligaments, and femoral head and neck pathology.

Return to Activity: As symptoms allow.

10.10 Hip Pointer

South Med J 1983;76:873

Cause: Contusion to ASIS due to direct blow.

Epidem: Most common in football, hockey, and other collision sports.

Pathophys: Soft tissue and bone bruising at the site of impact.

Sx: Pain and bruising following an appropriate mechanism.

Si:
- Tenderness at ASIS.
- Pain with hip abduction or flexion.

Crs: Symptoms generally resolve in 2-6 w.

Diff Dx:
- Trochanteric bursitis (see 10.8), snapping hip syndrome (see 10.9), hip pointer (see 10.10), neuropathies involving the lumbar nerve roots (L2-4) and branches of the iliohypogastric or subcostal nerves, sclerotomal irritation of lumbar facet joints and paraspinal ligaments, and femoral head and neck pathology.

X-ray: Plain radiographs to evaluate possible fracture of iliac apophysis.

Rx:
- Rest and protection.
- Ice early, heat in subacute phase.

Return to Activity: As symptoms allow.

Posterior Hip/Buttocks

10.11 Piriformis Syndrome

Orthopedics 1998;21:1133

Cause: Symptoms arise from muscle spasm, insertional inflammation, or by irritation of sciatic nerve.

Epidem: Most common in cyclists and roller sports, more common in females.

Pathophys:

- Piriformis muscle originates at the sacrum and inserts on the greater trochanter and functions in external rotation of the hip.
- The sciatic nerve lies deep to the muscle and may pass through the muscle belly in up to 15% of athletes.

Sx:

- Aching pain in buttocks often with sciatica.
- Worse with prolonged sitting or riding.

Si:

- Marked tenderness over gluteal prominence.
- Pain with resisted abduction and external rotation of the hip, and passive internal rotation of the hip (examined with the pt lying and knee in full extension).
- Normal neurologic examination, but positive straight leg raise.

Crs: Chronic, waxing, and waning symptoms.

Diff Dx:

- Ischial bursitis (see 10.12), sciatica (see 9.2), lumbar disc disease (see 9.2 and 9.4), and sacroilliac dysfunction (see 9.3).

X-ray:

- Non-indicated for piriformis syndrome.
- Lumbar spine x-ray and MRI may rule out lumbar DJD or disc disease as a cause of sciatica.

Rx:

- PRICEMM.
- Deep tissue massage.
- Physical therapy to improve flexibility and correct underlying SI dysfunction.
- Chiropractic or osteopathic treatments frequently helpful.

- Corticosteroid injection may be helpful but must be approached with caution.
- Padded seat for cyclist.

10.12 Ischiogluteal Bursitis (Weaver's Bottom)

Am Fam Phys 1996;53:2317

Cause: Inflammation of this bursa is associated with chronic and continuous direct stress.

Epidem: Occurs most frequently in sedentary occupations.

Pathophys: The bursa lies deep to the gluteus maximus over the ischial tuberosity.

Sx: Complain of pain in ischium with sitting and walking.

Si:
- Tenderness over the ischial tuberosity.
- Exacerbated by passive flexion and resisted extension of the hip.

Crs:
- Chronic pain.
- Symptoms usually relieved with treatment.

Diff Dx:
- Piriformis syndrome (see 10.11), sciatica (see 9.2), lumbar disc disease (see 9.2 and 9.4), and sacroilliac dysfunction (see 9.3).

X-ray: Negative.

Rx:
- PRICEMM.
- Rehabilitation through improving flexibility and strength.
- Lifestyle or occupational modification to decrease the direct pressure on this area.

- If vocational demands require continued sitting, a foam pad or air-filled "doughnut" to decrease direct pressure over the affected ischial tuberosity should be used.

Thigh

10.13 Muscle Strains

J Am Acad Orthop Sug 1998;6:237

Cause: Occurs due to a single macrotraumatic injury or from repetitive overuse.

Epidem: Hamstring muscle/tendon injuries are extremely common.

Pathophys: The most common site of injury is the musculotendinous junction.

Sx:
- The presenting symptoms depend on the mechanism of injury.
- Acute strains present with severe pain following a definable event, such as a sprint or jump.
- An overuse injury will have a gradual onset of pain, which eventually prevents running or other activities.

Si:
- Tenderness at the musculotendinous junction, which is made worse with active contraction of the muscle.
- Swelling, calor, and in the case of muscle tear, ecchymosis, and a palpable defect are often seen.

Crs:
- Acute injuries resolve in 1-4 w.
- Overuse injuries can result in chronic recurrent symptoms.

X-ray: MRI documents location and extent of injury, but seldom required.

Rx:
- Relative rest, avoiding activities which exacerbate the symptoms until the pain resolves, usually 1-4 w.
- An aggressive stretching program, aimed at the hamstrings, quadriceps, and calf, should be instituted as symptoms allow.
- The adjunctive use of NSAIDs, ice, ultrasound, and electrical stimulation are useful for pain relief.

10.14 Muscle Contusions

Am J Sports Med 1991;19:299

Cause: The usual mechanism is a direct blow.

Epidem: The most common examples in the hip and thigh region are quadriceps contusions and injuries to the ASIS (hip pointer).

Pathophys: Direct trauma results in bleeding and swelling into the muscle or periosteum.

Sx:
- Complaints of pain and bruising following appropriate mechanism.
- Pain with active contraction of affected muscle group.

Si:
- Localized tenderness, swelling, and ecchymosis at the site.
- Pain with passive stretch of affected muscle.
- Palpable muscle defect or bruise.

Crs: Full recovery is normal in 1-4 w.

X-ray: MRI can delineate any tear or defect in the muscle, but rarely necessary.

Rx:
- PRICEMM.
- For quadriceps contusion in the acute setting, an elastic wrap should be applied to the leg and calf with knee flexed 120° to

hold the quadriceps in a stretched position for 12-24 hr. This will limit the loss of flexibility in this muscle.

- These injuries should be treated with a gentle stretching program with a return to activity as soon as symptoms allow.

10.15 Myositis Ossificans

Orthop Rev 1992;21:1319

Cause: Myositis ossificans most commonly follows a quadriceps contusion or severe hamstring injury with deep tissue bleeding.

Epidem:
- Collision sports (football, hockey, rugby).
- Quad compartment and post thigh are most common but has been reported in many areas.

Pathophys: Represents metaplastic formation of bone in the muscle.
- Is most likely to arise following repetitive trauma.

Sx: History of substantial muscle injury, followed by persistent painful mass in area of trauma.

Si:
- Firm mass typically palpable.
- A gradual muscle contracture may occur with limited range of motion at the adjacent joints.

Crs: Bony mass develops 4-6 w following injury.

X-ray: Radiographs demonstrate early calcium deposition, followed by bone formation in the soft tissues.

Rx:
- Treatment of myositis ossificans includes a prevention of repetitive injury.
- Aggressive stretching and strengthening is advocated by some authors; others suggest absolute rest with early findings of MO.
- Surgical release of the mature ossificans sometimes required.

10.16 Avulsion Injuries

Skeletal Radiol 1994;23:85

Cause: Avulsion fractures about the pelvis occur following an acute, forceful contraction against fixed resistance.

Epidem: These are most common in the skeletally immature athlete. Several tendon insertion sites are commonly involved including:
- Sartorius avulsion from the anterior iliac crest (ASIS).
- Rectus femoris at the anterior inferior iliac spine.
- Hamstring origin at the ischium.
- Iliopsoas at the lesser trochanter.
- Piriformis at the greater trochanter.

Sx: Sudden pain at the insertion site with swelling, ecchymosis, and tenderness.

Si: Active muscle testing will significantly exacerbate the patient's pain.

X-ray: Radiographs are usually diagnostic for these injuries.

Rx:
- PRICEMM.
- Cautioned against challenging the effected muscle to the point of pain for 4-6 w.
- Structured flexibility and strengthening program should be instituted as soon as symptoms allow.
- Surgical treatment may be required with significant displacement of the avulsed segment in iliopsoas or ischial injuries.

Chapter 11
Knee

Acute Injuries

11.1 Anterior Cruciate Ligament (ACL)

Sports Med 2003;33:455; Am J Knee Surg 1998;11:128

Cause:
- Mechanism of injury is direct blow to the lateral, medial, or anterior aspects of the knee causing valgus or varus strain, twisting (rotational), or hyperextension.

Epidem:
- Varies by activity: alpine skiing, 7/1,000 skier days; collegiate football, 5/1,000 player days; general population, 3/1,000 knee injuries.
- Women appear to have increased risk in some sports compared with men. Thought to be related to increased Q angle (formed by the line from the ASIS to the center of the patella, and a line from the center of the patella to the tibial tubercle), narrower femoral notch, and smaller diameter ligament.

Pathophys:
- Major stabilizer preventing anterior translation of the tibia with respect to the femur, secondary rotational stabilizer.
- Injuries to other intra-articular structures (menisci, collateral ligaments) are commonly associated.

Sx:

- Patient typically describes a substantial trauma to the knee and often reports hearing or feeling a pop.
- Followed (within 2 hr) by a massive joint effusion (hemarthrosis).
- Pain is diffuse and typically related to bone bruising and/or meniscal injury.
- In chronic injuries, often complain of instability with quick turns or pivot movements.

Si:

- Acutely, substantial intra-articular effusion is palpable; joint line or posterior tenderness is common.
- Patency of neurovascular structures should be assessed.
- Lachman test: the patient is supine and relaxed, the knee is flexed to 20°, stabilize the distal femur with one hand while exerting an anteriorly directed force on the proximal tibia. Excessive anterior translation of the tibia when compared to the uninjured knee indicates laxity (Figure 11.1).
- Pivot shift: the patient is supine and the leg extended with the foot internally rotated, a valgus force is applied at the knee as the knee is slowly flexed. At approximately 30° a rotatory clunk will indicate a pos test.

Diff Dx:

- Other causes of hemarthrosis (fracture, PCL, MCL, LCL, patellar dislocation, meniscal tear).
- Other causes of instability (PCL, MCL, LCL, patellar dislocation).

Crs:

- Acute symptoms subside over 4-6 w; effusion may persist for 8-12 w.
- Instability and re-injury of intra-articular structures common.
- With recurrent instability, gradual degenerative disease is common.

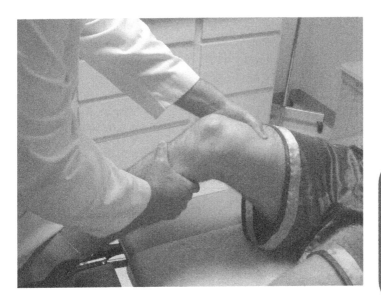

Figure 11.1 Lachman Test

X-ray:

- Radiographs will occasionally demonstrate a Segond lesion (avulsion fracture at the lateral proximal tibia).
- MRI is confirmatory, but not always necessary, however is useful to evaluate for other associated intra-articular injuries.

Rx:

- Initial: knee immobilizer for 24-72 hr with crutch ambulation. PRICEMM is useful for symptom relief. Structured therapy program should be instituted early to limit strength loss and maintain range of motion.
- Subacute: structured therapy including proprioception training and strengthening. Functional bracing for activities.

- Surgery: indication for surgery is persistent instability. Determinates include: age, chosen sport, level of participation, response to therapy. Surgery is usually delayed 2-6 w after injury.

Return to Activity:
- Nonoperative treatment, graded return to sport over 6-12 w.
- Surgical treatment, return to play 6-12 months following surgery.

11.2 Posterior Cruciate Injuries

Am J Sports Med 2004;32:361; Am J Knee Surg 1996;9:200

Cause:
- Direct blow to the anterior aspect of the knee (as in a motor vehicle accident), extreme flexion or anterior directed stress with the knee in full extension (usually results in combined ACL/PCL injury).

Epidem:
- Much less common than ACL injuries.
- Most common in football and hockey.
- NFL draftees have approximately 2% incidence.

Pathophys:
- Arises proximally on the medial femoral condyle in the intra-condylar notch. The fibers blend with the posterior capsular fibers at insertion on the proximal posterior tibia.
- The complex biomechanical architecture primarily functions to prevent posterior translation of the tibial with respect to the femur.
- The PCL also limits hyperextension and internal rotation.

Sx:
- Acute: pain in the posterior/lateral knee, swelling and occasionally instability with deceleration motions (as in walking down stairs).
- Chronic instability.

Si:
- Posterolateral tenderness, effusion. Positive instability testing.
- Posterior drawer sign: with the patient supine, flex the hip to 45° and the knee to 90° with the foot flat on the table; a posteriorly directed force is applied to the proximal anterior tibia. Increased translation indicates PCL injury.
- Sag sign: with the patient supine, the hips and knees are flexed to 90° with both feet supported above the table, a torn PCL will allow the tibial to translate posteriorly in this position in comparison to the uninjured knee.

Cmplc:
- Chronic instability leads to DJD.
- Instability can lead to damage to other intra-articular structures.

Diff Dx:
- Other causes of hemarthrosis (fracture, ACL, MCL, LCL, patellar dislocation, meniscal tear.
- Other causes of instability (ACL, MCL, LCL, patellar dislocation).

Crs: Instability may develop late (years after injury).

X-ray:
- Radiographs usually negative.
- MRI typically diagnostic.

Rx:
- Initial and nonoperative treatment as for ACL injuries.
- Reconstruction of PCL injuries is less common than for ACL tears, but may be indicated if instability persists following non-operative treatment.

KNEE

11.3 Meniscus Injuries

J Anat 1998;193:161; Am J Sports Med 2004;32:337

Cause:
- Twisting injury with the foot planted, valgus or varus strain, hyperextension, or hyperflexion.
- Often the trauma will appear minor or no specific event is recalled on history.

Epidem:
- Approximately 60/100,000 general population.
- Most common in cutting sports, football, soccer, basketball, wrestling.

Pathophys:
- Two "C" shaped fibrocartilagenous structures anchored via the capsule to the tibial plateau.
- They are thinner (and thus avascular) centrally, with the periphery relatively well vascularized.
- Function in both load sharing to dissipate forces on the proximal tibia, and in maintaining joint integrity.

Sx:
- An appropriate mechanism may be described, mild to moderate swelling, joint line pain, pain with flexion or extension, and a sensation of locking or catching within the knee joint.

Si:
- Effusion, joint line tenderness, and painful passive range of motion. Positive meniscal signs:
  - The Mcmurrays test: with the patient supine the hip is flexed to 90° and the knee maximally flexed, the examiner then internally or externally rotates the tibia and extends the knee while exerting a valgus or varus force respectively at the knee. A Mcmurrays test is positive if these maneuvers produce a painful pop.

- The Apley's compression test: with the patient prone the knee is flexed to 90° and a load is applied to the tibia while the tibia is internally and externally rotated; this will cause pain with a damaged meniscus.

Complc:
- Meniscal degeneration.
- Degenerative joint disease.
- Locked knee.

Diff Dx:
- Other causes of joint swelling (fracture, ligament injury, DJD).
- Other causes of locking or catching (patellar dysfunction).
- Other medial or lateral pain entities (ITB friction syndrome, bursitis).

Crs: Acute symptoms (pain with weight bearing, swelling, painful ROM) last 2-3 w with gradual improvement over 8-12 w.

X-ray:
- Plain radiographs are negative.
- MRI scan is useful for confirming diagnosis, but unnecessary if clinical evaluation conclusive.

Rx:
- Nonoperative treatment is effective in 50-75% of pts with an uncomplicated meniscal tear.
- Initially, PRICEMM measures with activity modification including short-term crutch use and limited walking for 3-5 d will reduce pain symptoms.
- Following the initial rest period, the patient should initiate exercise aimed at maintaining strength and flexibility while limiting pain. Alternate activities include cycling, walking, and pool running or swimming.
- As symptoms resolve, a gradual running program can be instituted with low intensity, short runs without hills or turns. Cutting and twisting activities should be avoided for 8-10 w.

KNEE

- If symptoms fail to resolve in 6-12 w, the pt should be referred for diagnostic imaging (MRI) or surgical evaluation.
- In a mechanically locked knee (ie, a loss of motion due to meniscal impingement) referral for urgent reduction or surgery should be arranged.

Return to Activity: As outlined above.

11.4 Patellar Dislocation and Subluxation

Acta Orthop Scand 1997;68:419

Cause:
- The most common mechanism is a twisting or valgus motion with a forceful quadriceps contraction.
- May be caused by direct blow to medial patella.

Epidem: Reported in a wide variety of sports. Most frequent in jumping and contact activities.

Pathophys:
- The patella usually dislocates laterally, over the femoral condyle.
- This displacement may be a true dislocation or may be partial which spontaneously reduces (patellar subluxation).
- Predisposing factors include quadriceps muscle imbalance (VMO hypoplasia with vastus lateralis hypertrophy), patella alta, hypoplastic femoral condyles, increased Q angle, and other functional malalignment.

Sx:
- Report a sensation of the lateral patellar displacement.
- In subluxation, the patella spontaneously reduces as the knee is extended.
- Substantial pain, locking, and swelling are common.

Si:
- If dislocation is seen acutely, the knee is held in flexion with the patella easily palpable on the lateral aspect of the joint.

- The orientation of the patella should be determined to plan reduction.
- Following subluxation a large effusion is common and the soft tissues medial to the patella (the retinaculum) will be tender to palpation.
- Lateral patellar pain is also common.
- Apprehension test (Figure 11.2): in patients with spontaneous reduction or subluxation, patellar stability is assessed by placing the patient supine with the knee flexed over the examiner's thigh (approximately 10°). The examiner applies pressure to the medial patella forcing it laterally; pain and increased motion are suggestive of patellar instability.

Crs:

- Dislocation requires reduction.
- Following reduction, pain at medial retinaculum and lateral patella subside over 4-8 w.

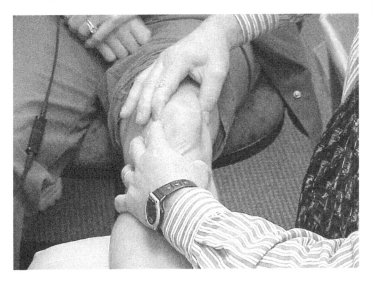

Figure 11.2 Patellar Apprehension Test

Complc:
- Patella fracture.
- Degenerative joint disease.

X-ray:
- Radiographs should be obtained to rule out evidence of fracture or loose body.
- MRI is useful to exclude other intra-articular injury.

Rx:
- If the pt presents with acute patellar dislocation, reduction can be attempted by extending the knee while applying gentle pressure to the lateral edge of the patella.
- Following the reduction, the knee should be immobilized for 6 w in full extension with a padded knee immobilizer or cylinder cast.
- These pts will require aggressive physical therapy to regain full function after prolonged immobilization.
- In subluxation without frank dislocation, short-term immobilization until pain resolves (2-4 w) followed by physical therapy aimed at VMO strengthening and improved flexibility will generally be effective (see 22.4).
- This is followed by the use of a patella brace (open patella knee sleeve) and activity modification as needed.
- Surgery may be required in pts with recurrent patellar dislocations.

Return to Activity:
- 2-8 w, depending on severity of symptoms and response to therapy.

11.5 Quadriceps/Patellar Tendon Rupture

Ortho Clin North Am 1992;23:613; J Am Acad Orthop Sug 2003;11:192

Cause: Most commonly injured through an eccentric overload event with a forceful quadriceps contraction in landing (deceleration), jumping (acceleration), or through a direct blow.

Epidem:
- Most frequent in sports with extreme eccentric overload (jumping, weight lifting, and football).
- Associated with chronic tendinitis and/or corticosteroid injections to the patellar tendon.

Pathophys:
- The extensor mechanism includes the quadriceps muscle group and linkage to the proximal tibia (quadriceps tendon-patella-patellar tendon-tibial tubercle).
- Disruption can occur at any point along this kinetic chain.

Sx:
- The pt will usually describe an appropriate mechanism.
- Painful swelling anteriorly.
- Weakness in standing or ambulation.

Si:
- Frequently a defect in the extensor mechanism can be palpated.
- Swelling, tenderness, and an intra-articular effusion are generally present.
- Extensor lag sign: pt will be unable to maintain knee extension against gravity or actively extend from a flexed position.

Crs: Requires surgical repair.

X-ray:
- Plain radiographs may demonstrate patellar fracture, tibial tubercle avulsion, or tendon avulsion from the patellar poles.
- MRI is very useful in localizing and grading severity of injury.

KNEE

Rx:
- Initial treatment is immobilization in full extension.
- Surgical consultation within 24-48 hr.

Return to Activity: 12-16 w following surgical repair and therapy.

11.6 Medial Collateral Ligament

Sports Med 1996;21:147

Cause: A valgus stress applied to the lateral knee either through direct blow or noncontact rotational stress.

Epidem: Common in cutting and contact sports, such as soccer, football, and basketball. Most common knee ligament injury in female alpine skiers.

Pathophys: These injuries are graded on a scale of 1 through 3. Grade 1 injury denotes a strain without disruption of the ligament (a simple stretch injury); grade 2 injury involves partial disruption of the ligament; and grade 3 injury is a complete disruption.

Sx:
- Pts will complain of medial joint pain following an appropriate mechanism.
- Pain will extend to distal medial femoral condyle or proximal tibia. Pain is worse in full extension or flexion beyond 90°.
- Initially, swelling may be minimal due to disruption of capsule. Swelling is common after the first 24 hr.
- In complete disruption, may experience symptoms of valgus instability.

Si:
- Medial joint line tenderness that extends above or below the joint to the origin or insertion of the ligament.
- Moderate effusion common.
- Passive range of motion is painful at full extension or flexion beyond 90°.

- Valgus stress test: with pt supine, the knee is flexed to 20°. A valgus strain is applied while maintaining a fulcrum at the lateral knee. This will produce pain at the medial knee and with a complete tear, medial joint space opening.
- Anterior drawer: the pt is supine with the knee flexed to 90° and the tibia placed in external rotation. With a complete tear, the medial tibial plateau will rotate anteriorly when an anteriorly directed force is applied to the posterior proximal tibia.

Crs:

- Grade 1 injury: return to play 1-2 w.
- Grade 2 injury: return to play in 3-6 w.
- Grade 3 injury: return to play in 6-12 w.

X-ray:

- Plain radiographs are nondiagnostic in MCL injuries; valgus stress radiographs will often document instability, but are not routinely obtained. MRI will often document location of injury and can distinguish grade 3 injuries from less severe strains. The main utility of MRI in these cases is to evaluate for associated injury to other structures.

Rx:

- Low-grade injuries: crutch ambulation, rest, ice, NSAIDs, and functional bracing with a full ROM to relieve acute symptoms.
- Rehabilitative exercises should be instituted as symptoms resolve. The pt should be started on alternative exercise activities, such as bicycling, as soon as possible, and resume running as symptoms allow. Advise the pt to run on flat surfaces avoiding any quick turns or cutting activities until symptoms completely resolve.
- Grade 3 injuries are treated as above except initial immobilization should restrict patient to 30° from full extension (extension block). This is maintained for 2-4 w.
- Functional rehabilitation including strengthening and flexibility work should be started as symptoms subside.

- MCL bracing should be maintained throughout rehabilitative process.
- With persistent instability or pain, further evaluation is indicated to rule out other intra-articular injury.
- Surgery may be required if instability persists following rehabilitation or if indicated for associated injuries to the ACL, LCL, or menisci.

Return to Activity:
- Low-grade injuries may return to activity in 1-2 w, if effectively braced.
- Higher-grade injuries, especially in contact sports, require 6-10 w to return to sport.

11.7 Lateral Collateral Ligament

Sports Med 1990;9:244

Cause:
- These injuries usually occur with a varus strain, twisting, or hyperextension injury.

Epidem:
- Less common than MCL injury.
- Common with other significant ligamentous injury of the knee.

Pathophys:
- Ligament arises on the lateral femoral condyle and inserts on the fibular head. It is a component of the arcuate complex serving to reinforce the posterior $1/3$ of the capsule and serves as a primary varus restraint.
- Complete LCL disruption is rarely an isolated injury, frequently associated with complete ACL tear, arcuate ligament complex injuries, and injury to other intra-articular structures.

Sx:

- These pts will complain of lateral joint pain with symptoms above or below the joint line at the insertion of the ligament.
- Pts may complain of instability with pivoting or twisting activities.
- Swelling and bruising are common.

Si:

- Tenderness at the lateral joint line with extension to the ligament insertion above or below the joint.
- Intra-articular effusion is common.
- Careful assessment of other intra-articular structures is key.
- Varus stress test: the knee is held at 20° flexion and a varus force is applied with the examiner's body while using the hand as a fulcrum on the medial joint space. This will produce pain or an opening in the joint. These injuries are graded 1-3 similarly to MCL injuries.
- Anterior drawer: the patient is supine with the knee flexed to 90° and the tibia placed in internal rotation. With a complete tear, the lateral tibial plateau will rotate anteriorly when an anteriorly directed force is applied to the posterior proximal tibia.
- Should be assessed for rotatory instability (see ACL/PCL).

Crs:

- Low-grade injury similar to low-grade MCL injury.
- Higher-grade injuries with instability often require surgery.

X-ray:

- Radiographs may demonstrate capsular avulsion injury.
- MRI typically diagnostic.

Rx:

- Low-grade strains without evidence of other injury can be managed in the same manner as an MCL injury.

- Injuries involving complete disruption of the LCL, posterolateral rotatory instability, or evidence of other intra-articular injury should be referred for orthopedic surgery evaluation.

Return to Activity:
- Low-grade injuries may return to activity in 1-2 w, if effectively braced.
- Higher-grade injuries, especially in contact sports or those requiring surgery, require significantly longer to return to sport.

Chronic Knee Problems

11.8 Retropatellar Knee Pain (Patellofemoral Pain)

Orthopedics 1997;20:148

Cause: Overuse syndrome in setting of knee malalignment.

Epidem: This is the most common cause of chronic anterior knee pain in the young athlete.

Pathophys:
- Etiologic factors are described as intrinsic, those related to anatomy, and extrinsic or external factors.
- Intrinsic factors include patellar malalignment (increased Q angle, patella alta or baja, lateral patellar tilt), quadriceps muscle imbalance, poor hamstring and quadriceps tendon flexibility, illiotibial band tightness, VMO hypoplasia, and foot biomechanics.
- Contributing extrinsic factors include inappropriate or overly worn footwear, precipitous changes in training volume, and poor training technique, to name a few.
- Symptoms arise from patellar chondral injury (chondomalacia patellae), synovial pinch, or synovitis.

Sx:
- Symptoms typically begin in adolescence often 30-60 d after changing activity.

- Pain is usually retro or peripatellar without associated joint line tenderness.
- Exacerbated by running, climbing stairs, or sitting with the knee flexed for extended periods of time.
- Subpatellar grinding sensation and snapping or popping with activity are common.
- Swelling is usually minimal.
- Pain related instability ("giving way") may occur.

Si:
- Peripatellar tenderness, mild swelling, and small joint effusion.
- Clinical signs of malalignment are common with a lateral shift of the patella with active extension, increased Q angle, positive Ober's test, and overpronated gait.
- Patellar grind: the pt lies supine with the knee flexed 10°, pressure is applied to the proximal patella or quadriceps tendon as the patient actively flexes the quadriceps. The test is considered pos if it produces pain.

Diff Dx:
- Plica syndrome (see 11.10), meniscal tear (11.3), patellar tendinitis, bursitis (prepatellar, pes anserine) (see 11.12), DJD.

Crs:
- Arises with new activity or change in training.
- Untreated, will commonly result in inability to participate.

X-ray:
- Lateralization of patella on AP view.
- Lateral patellar tilt on sunrise view.

Rx:
- Treatment goals are twofold: to provide symptom relief and to improve functional patellar alignment.
- PRICEMM provides a useful guide for symptom modifying measures.
- Pt should be educated regarding the etiology and contributing factors.

- An aggressive physical therapy program should include quadriceps, ITB, and hamstring stretching, and balanced quadriceps strengthening (with particular attention to VMO strengthening) (see 22.4).
- Typically 30-60 d is required, with specific limitations to running, jumping, and squatting activities.
- The use of an open patella knee sleeve or various taping techniques may also be helpful for symptom relief.
- The pt should be instructed on alternative activities such as cycling, swimming, or ski machine. These activities should be prescribed during the rehabilitative period.
- Occasionally, surgery may be useful in individuals with the more severe form (chondromalacia patellae). Pts with severe symptoms and clinical evidence of chondromalacia may be candidates for diagnostic arthroscopy and lateral release.

Return to Activity: As symptoms allow.

11.9 Tendinitis—Patellar or Quadriceps

Am J Knee Surg 1999;12:99

Cause:
- Precipitated by excessive jumping or running with similar underlying intrinsic and extrinsic factors as found in RPPS (malalignment, poor shoe wear, technical deficiencies).
- Due to the association with these activities, this injury is often referred to as "jumper's knee."

Epidem: Most common in repetitive eccentric overload sports, including basketball, volleyball, alpine skiing.

Pathophys:
- Symptoms are due to inflammation of the tendon, usually at the insertion on the inferior pole of the patella.
- Precipitated by eccentric overload

Sx:
- Anterior knee pain localized to the patellar or quadriceps tendon.
- Mild swelling, erythema, and warmth.
- Stiffness common after rest.

Si:
- Examination reveals tenderness and soft tissue swelling along the patellar tendon particularly at the inferior pole of the patella.
- Malalignment is typically seen with an increased Q angle, lateral patellar tracking, and weak ankle dorsiflexors.
- The posterior muscle/tendon chain and the quadriceps tendon are generally tight.

Diff Dx: RPPS (see 11.8), plica syndrome (see 11.10), meniscal tear (see 11.3), bursitis (prepatellar, pes anserine) (see 11.12), DJD.

Crs:
- Frequently results in chronic pain.
- Can contribute to patellar tendon rupture if untreated.

X-ray:
- Lateralization of patella on AP view.
- Lateral patellar tilt on sunrise view.

Rx:
- Directed towards symptom relief initially with activity modification, NSAIDs, ice, and elevation.
- Definitive therapy aims at correcting the functional malalignment and tightness through structured physical therapy.
- The pt should be advised to continue in alternative, non-painful activities while in rehabilitation.
- The infrapatellar strap has been advocated for symptom relief and may be useful in some individuals.

Return to Activity: As symptoms allow.

11.10 Medial Plica Syndrome

Am J Sports Med 1994;22:692

Cause: The plica may become inflamed either by acute compression of the patella or through repetitive extension/flexion activities.

Epidem: Synovial plica present in 20-60% of athletes.

Pathophys:
- The synovial plica is an embryologic remnant that arises at the medial lining of the suprapatellar pouch and attaches to the synovium beneath the infrapatellar fat pad.
- The medial edge of the plica protrudes from the medial joint in 20-50% of individuals.

Sx: Chronic anteromedial knee pain, which is worse with running or jumping activities.

Si:
- There may be mild soft tissue swelling.
- The plica is usually palpable along the medial patellofemoral joint, with the knee held in slight flexion and the tibia internally rotated.

Diff Dx: RPPS (see 11.8), tendinitis (see 11.9), meniscal tear (see 11.3), bursitis (prepatellar, pes anserine) (see 11.12), DJD.

Crs: Frequently arises from an acute traumatic event, then persists through repetitive motion injury.

X-ray: May show malalignment issues (patellar lateralization and tilt).

Rx:
- Activity modification and PRICEMM for symptom management.
- Flexibility exercises for the posterior chain and quadriceps group.
- Modification of functional malalignment, as outlined for RPPS, should also be done if malalignment is present (see 22.4).

- Surgical treatment for this is common, but has mixed results.
- Anti-inflammatory steroid injection often helpful for symptom management. Triamcinolone (20-40 mg) with 2-3 cc of lidocaine is injected using sterile technique into the plica and surrounding soft tissue. Care must be taken not to inject anteriorly in the area of the patellar tendon.

Return to Activity: As symptoms allow.

11.11 Prepatellar Bursitis (Housemaid's Knee, Coal Miner's Knee)

Am Fam Phys 1996;53:2317

Cause: This is usually associated with trauma, either chronic, as with repetitive kneeling (housemaid's knee) or an acute injury, such as a blow to the knee.

Epidem: The prepatellar bursa is one of the most common sites for septic bursitis.

Pathophys:
- Swelling in the bursa between the patella and skin.
- May be infectious or inflammatory.

Sx:
- Anterior knee pain, stiffness, pain with motion.
- Systemic signs of infection: fevers, chills, malaise.

Si:
- Swelling anterior to the patella.
- Infection should be considered if there is evidence of injury to the skin overlying the bursa.
- Other frequent findings with infectious bursitis include increased warmth, redness, severe tenderness, lymphadenitis, cellulitis, and fever.

Diff Dx:
- RPPS (see 11.8), patellar tendinitis (see 11.9), plica syndrome (see 11.10).

Crs: Infectious bursitis may involve intra-articular knee if untreated.

X-ray: Negative.

Rx:

- Aspiration should always be done if there is suspicion of an infection. This is done by first anesthetizing the skin with 1% lidocaine. A 22-gauge needle is inserted into the bursa under sterile conditions and the contents of the bursae aspirated using a 30-cc syringe.
- The aspirate should be sent for analysis including: appearance, cell count, gram stain, culture, and microscopy. Approximately 90% of these infections are due to *Staphylococcus aureus* or *S. epidermidis* and 9% to streptococcal species. Infectious bursitis requires drainage followed by antibiotic therapy.
- Pending culture results penicillinase resistant synthetic penicillins (dicloxacillin 500 mg qid/d), or first-generation cephalosporin (cephradine 500 mg qid/d) should be started.
- If septic arthritis is suspected, intra-articular aspiration should be performed and referral for arthroscopic surgery if aspirate confirms diagnosis.
- In nonseptic cases, treatment follows the general outline described previously.
- Wrapping the knee with an elastic bandage or padding for protection against further injury are helpful.

Return to Activity: As symptoms allow.

11.12 Pes Anserine Bursitis

Am Fam Phys 1996;53:2317

Cause: Direct blow to bursa or repetitive use of medial hamstring.

Epidem: Most common in collision sports and in older athletes with DJD of knee.

Pathophys: The pes anserine bursa lies behind the medial hamstring (formed by the tendons of the sartorius, gracilis, and semitendinosus [SGT] muscles).

Sx: Pain and tenderness over the anteromedial aspect of the proximal tibia, 4-5 cm below the joint line, which is exacerbated by active flexion of the knee.

Si:

- Examination reveals swelling over the anteromedial tibia just proximal to the insertion of the SGT tendons, which can be mistaken for a cyst or mass.
- The tenderness may track along the SGT tendons indicating an associated tendinitis.
- There is often evidence of patellar malalignment, as well as poor flexibility particularly in the hamstrings and quadriceps tendons.

Crs: Often chronic pain if untreated.

X-ray: Typically negative.

Rx:

- Treatment follows the general PRICEMM guidelines.
- Injected corticosteroids are very useful, however care must be taken not to inject the patellar tendons.
- Particular attention should be given to stretching the hamstrings, quadriceps, and Achilles tendons.

Return to Activity: As symptoms allow.

11.13 Popliteal (Baker's) Cysts

Am Fam Phys 1996;53:2317

Cause: Posterior knee swelling related to intra-articular effusion.

Epidem: Seen most commonly in association with chronic meniscal disease or degenerative joint disease.

Pathophys:
- Popliteal (Baker's) cysts usually arise from an intra-articular effusion.
- Swelling of the medial gastrocnemius or semimembranosus bursae may also cause a painful popliteal cyst.
- Popliteal cysts usually result from a significant intra-articular knee injury, osteoarthritis, rheumatoid arthritis, and less commonly gouty arthritis.

Sx: Symptoms include painful local swelling or popliteal mass that worsens with walking, jumping, or squatting.

Si:
- Physical exam will usually demonstrate a tender mass in the popliteal fossa.
- A careful examination of the knee must be done to rule out an associated internal derangement.

Diff Dx: Hamstring or popliteal tendinitis, meniscal tear (see 11.3), internal derangement, DVT.

Crs: Chronic intermittent posterior knee pain.

X-ray:
- Plain radiographs may demonstrate degenerative joint disease.
- Ultrasound or MRI are useful to differentiate an isolated semimembranosus bursa which communicates with the joint from a synovial hernia related to intra-articular pathology.

Rx:
- Treatment in adults should address the underlying cause of joint effusion (meniscal tear, DJD, etc).
- In children, popliteal cysts frequently are associated with intra-articular pathology and further workup by imaging studies is indicated.
- Intra-articular corticosteroid injection is often effective to alleviate swelling and symptoms temporarily.

Return to Activity: As symptoms allow.

11.14 Iliotibial Band Friction Syndrome (ITBFS)

Med Sci Sports Exerc 1995;27:951

Cause: Tightness in the ITB leads to friction irritation at the lateral femoral condyle resulting in inflammation and pain.

Epidem: Common in runners, dancers, and cross-country skiers

Pathophys:
- The iliotibial band (ITB) arises from the tensor fascialata muscle in the lateral buttocks, and runs along the lateral leg to its insertion at Gerdes tubercle on the anterolateral tibia.
- Predisposing factors include genu varum, leg length discrepancy, excessive foot pronation, as well as running on sloped surfaces, such as the cambered surface of a road.

Sx:
- These patients complain of lateral knee pain that is worse with activities such as running, jumping, and squatting.
- Character of pain frequently described as aching.

Si:
- Marked tenderness and swelling along the distal course of the ITB as it crosses the femoral condyle.
- Ober's sign: the patient is placed on his or her side and both hips flexed 90° with the knees flexed to 90°. The free leg is then maximally extended. Tightness in the ITB is demonstrated if the knee does not fall to the table.

Diff Dx: Lateral meniscal tear (see 11.3), lateral collateral ligament tear (see 11.7).

Crs: Acute irritation often becomes chronic pain if left untreated.

X-ray:
- X-ray negative.
- MRI may demonstrate effusion between ITB and lat femoral condyle.

KNEE

Rx:

- Pain relief and anti-inflammatory measures follow the general guidelines of PRICEMM.
- Corticosteroid injection (triamcinolone 40 mg or betamethasone 6 mg) is useful for symptom relief. The tender area is identified (usually at the lateral femoral condyle) and the steroid is injected beneath the ITB under sterile technique. Typically 2-3 cc of lidocaine is mixed with the steroid to provide immediate relief.
- Physical therapy is directed at improving ITB flexibility through stretching exercise and hip abductor strengthening (see 22.4).
- Treatment should also address any foot biomechanical issues and underlying sacroiliac dysfunction.

Return to Activity: As symptoms allow.

Chapter 12

Leg Problems

12.1 Stress Fractures

Clin Sports Med 1997;l6:259; Med Sci Sports Exerc 2000;32:S15; Clin J Sp Med 1991;1:115; Clin Sports Med 2004;23:55

Cause: Most commonly due to overuse injuries in context of sporting activity with repetitive or high impact training; less commonly seen in overuse or normal activity in context of an athlete with poor bone quality. Increase in running mileage or intensity, change in training shoes or poor training shoes, change to a harder or different running surface; most commonly occur in the proximal ⅔ of the tibia (Am J Sports Med 1987;15:46)

Epidem: Runners, sports involving running, military recruits; incidence higher in women, especially in women with irregular menses.

Pathophys:
- Risk factors: high impact activities, *pes planus* (flat foot), *pes cavus* (high-arched foot), low bone mineral density, limb length discrepancy, poor nutrition or eating disorders, menstrual irregularities.
- Imbalance between bone resorption and bone deposition during host bone response to stress.
- Microfractures progress to clinical stress fractures in the setting of continuing abusive activity and inadequate rest.

Sx: History of recent increase in duration, intensity or frequency of activity; dull or sharp pain, commonly in the proximal anterior tibia. Initially present after activity, progressing to pain during activity, then pain preventing activity; if pain is in the distal lateral aspect of leg, a fibular stress fracture may be present, (see 13.11); swelling may accompany stress fractures.

Si: Exam may be normal if patient is asymptomatic during inactivity; tenderness over the tibia or fibula, localized to an area less than 5 cm in diameter, is very suggestive of a stress fracture. Pain may be elicited by percussion or vibration proximal or distal to site of injury.

Cmplc: Progression to complete fracture, nonunion of fracture, displacement of fracture, chronic disabling leg pain. Athletes with stress fracture in the anterior central third of the tibia are very slow to heal and have a high risk of progression to complete fracture.

Diff Dx: MTSS (see 12.4), tibialis posterior syndrome, exertional compartment syndrome (see 12.2), fascial hernia, bone tumors.

X-ray:
- X-rays may appear normal in acute phase (as many as 50%).
- AP and lateral radiographs may show stress fractures that have been symptomatic for more than 3 w.
- Beware the anterior cortical tibial "dreaded black line" ("DBL," horizontal radiolucent line in anterior tibial cortex denoting chronic injuries and/or high likelihood of progression; if + DBL, refer to orthopedic surgery).
- Focal periosteal thickening or bony radiodensity may be seen in later phases; actual fracture line is rarely seen.
- If plain films negative and suspicion is still high, consider bone scan, MRI or CT.
- Bone scan will be positive 3-5 d after the onset of pain.

Rx: Stop pain-producing activities (including weight bearing if injury has progressed); modified weight bearing until no pain with ambulation; start RICE therapy; NSAIDs as needed; physical therapy for range of motion, strengthening and proprioceptive rehab once pain free. If able to perform pain free, cycling or swimming may be done to maintain fitness; healing time is 4-6 w for noncomplicated stress fractures. Consider diagnostic workup for osteoporosis/osteopenia or eating disorder and treat as indicated. If fails conservative treatment or becomes a chronic problem, refer to orthopedic surgery for possible operative fixation.

Return to Activity: Should be gradual; use of pneumatic leg braces has been shown in a small study to reduce healing time by up to several w (Am J Sports Med 1987;15:86).

12.2 Exertional Compartment Syndrome (ECS)

Orthop Rev 1994; 23:219-226; Med Sci Sports Exerc 2000;32:S4; Clin Sport Med 2004;23:55

Cause: Overuse injury in runners from impact activities.

Epidem: Runners, endurance athletes in sports requiring running; 14% of patients with lower leg pain; most commonly in anterior compartment (45%).

Pathophys:
- Exercise-induced soft tissue swelling in the limited volume of the fascial compartments produce ischemia.
- The compartments most frequently affected by ECS are the anterior, followed by the deep posterior, lateral, posterior tibial, and superficial posterior (see Table 12.1).

Sx:
- Exercise-induced aching, squeezing, or sharp pain in the anterior leg, exacerbated by increasing activity intensity or duration, and relieved by rest (may take several hr to resolve completely); symptoms that occur at rest more consistent with nerve entrapment syndromes (see Diff Dx).
- May be bilateral (75-90%).
- Pain often recurs at the same distance while running.

Table 12.1　Four Fascial Compartments of the Leg

Compartment	Muscles	Nerve	Sensory Area
Lateral	Peroneus brevis and longus	Superficial peroneal nerve	Dorsal foot
Anterior	Tibialis ant, Ext digitorum, and Hallucis	Deep peroneal nerve	Dorsal 1st and 2nd web space
Deep posterior	Flexor digit/hallux, posterior tibialis	Tibial nerve	Plantar foot
Superficial posterior	Soleus, gastrocnemius	Sural nerve	Lateral foot

- May have muscle or nerve dysfunction in the affected compartment (eg, numbness and tingling), most commonly the anterior or lateral compartments.
- Anterior leg may be diffusely swollen and described as "tense" (Sports Injuries, Diagnosis and Management. Philadelphia: WB Saunders Company, 1999:350).

Si: Examining immediately after exercise is more useful than at rest:
- Tenderness over the involved compartment.
- Fascial herniae are present in up to 46% of cases.
- Neurovascular exam is commonly normal, however, paresthesia may be present in affected legs; if the anterior compartment is affected, slight foot drop may be present, as well as decreased sensation in the first web space of the foot.
- Diagnosis is confirmed by measuring pre-exercise and post-exercise intracompartmental pressures; the necessary equipment is currently available in kit form.
- The American Academy of Orthopedic Surgeons has published the following diagnostic standards:
  1. Resting pressure exceeding 15 mm Hg before exercise.
  2. 1 min (or 5 min) postexercise pressure exceeding 30 mm Hg (or 20 mm Hg, respectively).

Cmple: Chronic leg pain; progression of neurovascular deficit.

Diff Dx: MTSS (see 12.4), stress fracture (see 12.1); popliteal artery entrapment (see 12.5), claudication, nerve entrapment syndrome.

X-ray: R/o stress fx; consider bone scan in refractory cases.

Rx:
- Nonoperative treatment is cessation or reduction of running (or aggravating activity).
- Cross training may be attempted.
- Operative treatment consists of fasciotomy of all affected compartments, with good overall results and return to full activity at 1-mo post surgery.

12.3 Tennis Leg (Gastrocnemius Tear)

Ankle 1985;5:186; Manual Sports Med 1998:460

Cause: Partial or total rupture of the medial head of the gastrocnemius muscle (aka gastroc).

Epidem: Common muscle injury in men older than 40 y/o participating in racquet sports, alpine skiing, jumping, and running; "weekend warrior": intermittently active athletes; occurs twice as frequently in men.

Pathophys: Partial tear most commonly at the musculotendinous junction of the medial belly of the gastrocnemius muscle; injury occurs with the knee fully extended and the ankle maximally dorsiflexed.

Sx: Sudden sharp pain in midposteromedial leg leading to an obligate immediate stop of sport activity. May report feeling that the back of the leg was hit; may hear or feel a "pop"; intense pain and swelling develop within 24 hr after injury, especially with walking; may be associated with prodromal ache or stiffness.

LEG PROBLEMS

Si: Tenderness at musculotendinous junction of medial gastroc with local pressure, passive ankle dorsiflexion, or active plantar flexion of the ankle; local defect can be palpated for a few hours post-injury; substantial, asymmetric swelling immediately and ecchymosis within 1-2 d.

Cmplc: Deep-vein thrombosis (DVT) secondary to extrinsic compression and immobilization; posterior compartment syndrome.

Diff Dx: Deep-vein thrombosis (Clin Sports Med 1997;16:475); Baker's cyst rupture, plantaris tendon rupture, compartment syndrome, popliteal artery entrapment (see 12.5).

X-ray: Ultrasonography is able to demonstrate the size of the lesion; plain films helpful only if fracture is suspected; MRI may also be helpful; Doppler sonogram if suspicious for DVT.

Rx:
- Rest, ice, elevation for the first 48 hr, with crutches for ambulating, as indicated.
- Short use of a ROM or CAM walker for immobilization in more severe cases.
- Neoprene sleeve for muscle support.
- Passive then active stretching of calf by 2 w.
- Heel lift or pad may make walking more comfortable until calf is able to stretch.

Return to Activity: Gradual return to activity when walking pain free; recovery time generally 4-12 w; full activity when 90% of normal strength is recovered.

12.4 Medial Tibial Stress Syndrome (MTSS, Shin Splints or Periostalgia)

Am J Sports Med 1985;13:398; Med Sci Sport Exerc 2000;32:S27; Clin J Sport Med 1995;5:53

Cause: Overuse injury caused by running in a deconditioned athlete, or sudden increase in intensity of training.

Epidem: Runners, jumpers, and participants in sports requiring running; 10-15% of all running injuries.

Pathophys:

- Has been attributed to stress along medial fascial insertion of the soleus muscle (soleus bridge) on the posteromedial border of middle and distal thirds of the tibia, causing myositis, fasciitis, and periostitis.
- Some have implicated the posterior tibialis or flexor digitorum longus (FDL).
- Excessive foot pronation has been implicated; the athlete is forced to pronate to accommodate for gastroc-soleus inflexibility.

Sx:

- History of recent changes in pattern, frequency or intensity of activity; poor fitting or worn shoes are major risk factors.
- Pain along the posteromedial border of the distal tibia, induced by exercise and relieved by rest.
- Initially pain is after activity.
- Pain at the start of activity, relieved during activity and returning after activity is consistent with MTSS
- Pain with resisted plantar flexion and inversion.
- Can be graded based on relation of symptoms to activity:
  Grade 1: Symptoms occur at start of activity, decrease during activity, or develop at the end of activity.
  Grade 2: Symptoms occur during activity with late onset.
  Grade 3: Symptoms during activity with early onset, persist throughout activity.
  Grade 4: Symptoms limit the quality or quantity of training.
  Grade 5: Symptoms prevent training.

Si: Exquisite tenderness along the posteromedial border of the distal third to the tibia; pain with standing on toes; pronated feet are a common finding; pain with passive ankle dorsiflexion or active ankle plantar flexion.

Cmplc: Chronic leg pain and poor performance.

Diff Dx: Exertional compartment syndrome of the deep posterior compartment (see 12.2), stress fracture (see 12.1), tumor, peroneal nerve entrapment, DVT, tennis leg (see 12.3), claudication, popliteal artery entrapment (see 12.5).

X-ray:
- Radiographs usually normal; posterior cortical hypertrophy, periosteal thickening, or cortical defects may be seen.
- Longitudinally oriented *diffuse* uptake involving one-third or more of the length of the bone are present on triple-phase bone scan (only on the delayed phase in MTSS: stress fractures will have more *focal* uptake in all 3 phases).

Rx:
- Rest for 1 w, with a very gradual return to full activity.
- Excessive pronators will benefit from fitted orthotics.
- Gastroc-soleus stretching.
- Other modalities, including NSAIDs, icing, crutches, steroids, etc, have not been shown to decrease healing time over rest alone.
- Cross training to maintain fitness (eg, swimming, water running, etc), and proprioceptive training once pain free, may be considered after 1-2 w of rest.

12.5 Vascular Causes of Exertional Leg Pain (Peripheral Vascular Disease, Popliteal Artery Entrapment, Adductor Canal Outlet Syndrome, Vasculitis, Deep Venous Thrombosis, Atherosclerosis, Adventitial Cystic Disease)

Curr Sports Med Rep 2004;3:67; Phy Sportsmed 2001;29:35; Phy Sportsmed 2002;30:23

Cause: Varies depending on which vascular cause, leading to impedance in blood flow to compartmental muscles.

Epidem: Rare, but important cause of exertional leg pain (ELP); those with peripheral vascular disease (PVD) are usually age 40-60 y/o; popliteal artery entrapment syndrome is seen in younger patients. 10-15% of patients with popliteal artery entrapment may have associated venous compression; M>F.

Pathophys:

- Pathophysiology depends on the vascular cause, all with a common mechanism of impeded arterial blood flow to compartmental muscles either due to intravascular causes (thromboses, atherosclerotic plaques, inflammation in the vascular walls) or dynamic, extravascular impingement/entrapment of blood vessels; popliteal artery entrapment may occur at origin of medial head of gastroc or plantaris muscles; or as a result of an aberrant vessel course.
- Risk factors include any hypercoagulable state and traditional cardiac risk factors (hypertension, diabetes, smoking, hyperlipidemia).

Sx:

- Poorly localized, crampy, achy leg pain; symptoms absent at rest, increases with exercise/activity. Pt may describe a consistent distance at which symptoms occur; may mimic exertional compartment syndrome (ECS; see 12.2).
- Look for the "5 Ps:" pain, pallor, paralysis, paraesthesia, pulselessness.
- Differences between ECS and vascular causes of ELP:
  - ECS: pain related to volume, amount or duration of activity, and persists for 30 min postexercise, with tight compartments on palpation.
  - Vascular ELP: pain associated with intensity and abates with stopping the activity.

Si: Exam may be normal at rest: consider exercise-stressing the pt before a repeat exam; include thorough neurovascular exam. May have posterior leg tenderness; ABI may be abnormal (in popliteal artery entrapment, ABI may be normal at rest).

Cmplc: Chronic leg pain, poor performance, limb ischemia, and possibly necrosis.

Diff Dx: Exertional compartment syndrome of the deep posterior compartment (see 12.2), stress fracture (see 12.1), tumor, nerve entrapment, tennis leg (see 12.3).

X-ray:

- All imaging studies should be performed with the knee extended, and with the ankle both dorsiflexed and plantar flexed.
- Arterial and venous Doppler ultrasound, MRI / MRA, angiography; consider a hypercoagulability workup, EKG, and/or echocardiogram.

Rx:

- Activity modification, smoking cessation, and addressing other modifiable risk factors.
- Consider referral to vascular surgery or hematology as indicated; other consultants may also be helpful.
- Treatment of underlying cause (eg, pletal, anticoagulation, stents, bypass).
- Return to play decisions should be made on a case-by-case basis, considering the risks of anticoagulation therapy as indicated (eg, consider avoiding contact sports due to bleeding risks).

Chapter 13

Ankle Injuries

Acute Injuries

13.1 Lateral Ankle Sprain

Clin Sports Med 1997;16:433; Phy Sportsmed 1993;21:123; Phy
    Sportsmed 1998; 26:29; Med Sci Sports Exerc 1999;31:S429

Cause: Excessive, rapid ankle inversion; the majority of ankle sprains
    involve the anterior talofibular ligament.

Epidem: Most common injury in athletics; 85% of all ankle injuries
    are sprains, more than 4 × as frequent than medial ankle sprains;
    85% are lateral and 85% involve the ATFL.

Pathophys: Inversion or an internal rotation force to a plantar-flexed
    ankle, which may result in partial or complete disruption of the
    lateral ligamentous complex; (anterior talofibular [ATFL], calca-
    neofibular [CFL], and, much less commonly, the posterior
    talofibular ligaments [PTFL]).

Sx: The pt may appreciate a "tear" or "pop" at the time of injury,
    which may indicate a complete tear; the pain is intense and lo-
    calized to the lateral ankle, often anterior or inferior to the lat-
    eral malleolus; the pain may initially improve in the first few
    hours, only to return with the presence of increased swelling;
    normal ROM is dorsiflexion (DF) 15-20°, plantar flexion (PF)
    50°, eversion (Ev), inversion (Inv).

Si:

- May have antalgic gait or other gait abnormalities.
- Tenderness to palpation (TTP) with or without swelling over ATFL, CFL, or PTFL.
- Ecchymosis over lateral ankle.
- Decreased active ROM.
- Access sensation in the distribution of the deep peroneal nerve (first webbed space of the foot).
- Access motor function and presence of dorsalis pedis and posterior tibial pulses.
- Tibiofibular squeeze test to assess for syndesmotic injury (see 14.4).
- May have pos Talar tilt test:
  - Performed with the pt seated and with the ankle in 10° of plantar flexion.
  - Stabilize the medial aspect of the distal part of the leg, just proximal to the medial malleolus, with one hand and apply an inversion force slowly to the hindfoot with the other hand; the affected side is compared against the normal side; if the talus gaps and rocks open this indicates laxity of the ATFL.
- May have pos anterior drawer test:
  - Performed with the foot in 10° of plantar flexion: tests for anterolateral rotatory instability due to anterior talofibular ligament instability.
  - Stabilize the distal part of the leg with one hand and apply an anterior force with the other hand on the heel, and attempt to subluxate the talus anteriorly from beneath the tibia.
  - The affected ankle is compared to the pt's normal ankle.
  - Alternative modified anterior drawer test (Figure 13.1) may be performed by having the pt rest each foot on the examining table with the knees bent at 90°; the examiner then stabilizes the foot on the exam table and provides a posterior

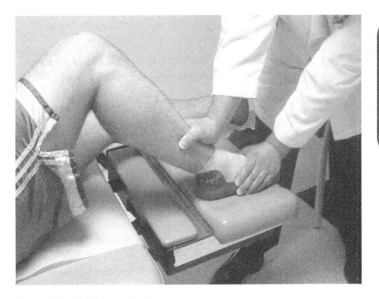

Figure 13.1 Modified anterior drawer test

force on the distal tibia and estimating the degree of posterior displacement of the tibia on the talus (anterior drawer).
- Talar tilt and anterior drawer tests may be difficult to perform in acute setting.
- Grading sprains:
  Grade I: mild stretching of the fibers within the ligament, but produce no evidence of laxity; disability 1-2 wk.
  Grade II: partial tear of ATFL and CFL with mild laxity, but good overall stability; disability 2-4 wks.
  Grade III: complete rupture of ATFL and CFL and cause unstable joint; associated with peroneal nerve damage; disability 2-6 mo.

Cmplc: Traction injuries of the peroneal and posterior tibial nerves can occur in severe injuries.

Diff Dx: Peroneal compartment syndrome, chronic syndesmotic injury (see 13.4), peroneal tendon subluxation (see 13.3), talar dome lesion (see 13.5), ankle fracture, Achilles tendon rupture (see 13.6), midfoot injury (see 14.18), lateral process fracture of the talus (prevalent in snowboarders, poorly visible on x-ray, CT if suspect).

X-ray:
- To rule out fracture or syndesmotic injury.
- Radiographic assessment of the syndesmosis: one of the more challenging and important tasks that the clinician must perform is to rule out an injury to the syndesmosis; the mortise and AP views must be utilized to review the criteria for diagnosing injury to the syndesmosis.
- Standard: anteroposterior (AP), lateral, and mortise views.
- Consider foot and leg films when clinically indicated.
- The radiographs should be evaluated for:
    1. The presence or absence of a medial malleolar fracture or widening of the space between the medial malleolus and the talus (aka medial clear space).
    2. The presence or absence of a fibular fracture, its relationship to the tibial plafond (ie, at, above or below), and the orientation of the fracture (ie, transverse, oblique or comminuted).
    3. Displacement of the distal tibiofibular joint (to assess competency of the syndesmosis; aka tibiofibular overlap).
    4. Displacement of the talus from its normal anatomic position beneath the tibia (aka: talar tilt; not the same as talar tilt test).
- Ottawa Rules: a decision protocol designed to avoid obtaining films on all ankle injuries by identifying patients at negligible

risk for fracture; 97%+ sensitivity for ruling out a fracture, but only a 31-63% specificity for ruling in fractures (Jama 1993;269:1127); essentially an ankle x-ray series is necessary only if there is pain near the malleoli and any of these findings:

- Inability to bear weight both immediately and in the emergency room (4 steps); or
- Bone tenderness at the posterior edge or posterior tip of either malleolus.

Rx: Refer to orthopedic surgeon if tibiofibular overlap is > 10 mm, there is > 2 mm difference between medial and lateral talar tilts, medial clear space is > 2 mm greater than superior, all medial and displaced lateral malleolar fractures, and lateral malleolar fracture > 2 mm displacement; consider referral for Grade III injuries; early protected mobilization and functional rehabilitation for all grades of sprain.

Ankle Rehabilitation:

Phase I: (Immediate postinjury) PRICEMM and early motion:

- Use crutches or cane if unable to walk without limp; emphasize normal heel-toe gait with progressive wt-bearing over 1-5 d
- PRICEMM:

Protect from further damage: ankle brace to limit inversion and eversion; Grade II sprains may require a short period of immobilization with a posterior splint or short leg cast; Grade III sprains may require up to 6-8 wks of immobilization.

Relative rest: limit activity; avoid abusing activity.

Ice: apply for 20 min at least 3-4 × per d for first 24-48 hr.

Compression: wrap ankle with ace wrap or ankle brace to control swelling; horseshoe felt around lateral malleolus may improve effectiveness of compression wraps.

Elevate: keep leg above heart as much as possible to help control swelling.

Medications: large-scale studies have demonstrated that non-steroidal anti-inflammatory drug (NSAID) used post-injury resulted in reduced subject pain, time lost from training, cost of treatment and increased exercise endurance; however, NSAID use was also associated with increased ligament laxity, decreased range-of-motion, and increased swelling; it is possible that the analgesic effects allow athletes to resume training prematurely (Am J Sports Med 1997;25:544); if NSAIDs are used, consider starting 48 hr postinjury to decrease risk of increased bleeding at injury site; acetaminophen for pain, as needed.

Modalities: physical therapy (electric-stim or ultrasound).

- Ice bath followed by stationary bike: immerse foot in ice bucket until foot is numb, and then ride bike until numbness wears off; repeat 4 ×.
- ROM exercise: write the capital letters of the alphabet with the big toe by moving at the ankle; only move to the point of stretching.

Phase II: Begin as soon as one can tolerate the listed activity without compensation (see 22.5):

- Stationary bike.
- Range-of-motion exercise (DF, PF, eversion, inversion).
- Balance and proprioception exercises: BAPS, foam roller balance.
- Theraband exercises: loop Theraband or surgical tubing around forefoot, hold proximal ends in hands; invert and evert against resistance.
- Heel raises and Achilles stretching: raise up on the balls of both feet, lifting the heels off the door; lower the heels slowly; repeat 30 repetitions; when stronger, raise up on strong foot, lower with only the injured foot.
- Contrast bath: 20 min.

Phase III: Begin when able to walk without limp:
- Add stairmaster, slide board, squats, and lunges.
- Balance and proprioception exercises: stand on effected leg on mini-trampoline; close eyes for 20 sec (go ahead and try it while healthy—it is an ankle workout); repeat 6 ×; stand on affected leg on mini-trampoline, play catch with a 1-2 kg medicine ball (or any ball); a useful alternative to a mini-trampoline is to use a folded towel on a hardwood floor.
- Ice ankle after exercise for 20 min.

Phase IV:
- Gradual return to jogging.
- Jump rope.
- Dot jumping, agility drills, balance and proprioception exercises (see above).
- Ice, as needed.
- Consider ankle brace for return to full activity.
- Progression from phase to phase is dependent upon individual progression, NOT time.

Prevention: Most common risk factor for ankle sprain is a history of previous sprain; complete supervised rehabilitation should be completed before return to practice; athletes suffering a moderate or severe sprain should wear an appropriate brace for at least 6 mo; properly fitting braces or correctly applied tape does not interfere with athletic performance; ankle taping provides effective support for less than 20 min of exercise, however it may help provide additional proprioception via the skin and reduce injury; lace-up braces and stirrup-style braces offer longer lasting support; ankle strengthening and proprioception training are the most effective form of prevention (Am J Sports Med 1999;277:573).
- Failure to improve in a reasonable time period of treatment may warrant a reconsideration of other diagnoses (see Diff Dx

and Chronic Ankle Injuries, see 13.8, 13.9, and 13.10) and possible referral for surgical evaluation.

Return to Activity:
- Normal range of motion.
- 85% of pre-injury strength.
- Minimal swelling.
- No pain with ADLs.
- Pain-free execution of functional drills such as hopping on injured leg or sprinting tight figure-eight pattern.
- Good proprioception as demonstrated by ability to single-leg stand with eyes closed for 25-30 sec.

13.2 Medial Ankle Sprain

J Emerg Med 1999;17:651; Clin Sports Med 1997;16:435

Cause: Excessive, rapid ankle eversion leading to injury of the deltoid ligament of the ankle.

Epidem: Less than 10% of ankle sprains; isolated deltoid injuries are far less common than lateral ankle sprains (see 14.1).

Pathophys: Pronation, abduction, external rotation, and/or eversion to the abducted foot, resulting in partial or complete disruption of the medial (aka, deltoid) ligamentous complex; superficial deltoid ligaments (tibionavicular, calcaneotibial / sustentacular, and posterior talotibial ligaments); deep deltoid ligaments (deep anterior talotibial, deep posterior talotibial ligaments); anterior fibers tear more frequently; deltoid ligament injuries less common and usually more severe than lateral ankle injuries; often associated with injuries to the fibula and lateral ligaments (see 13.1).

Sx: A "tearing" or "popping" sensation at the time of injury may indicate a complete tear; pain localized to medial ankle, often inferior to medial malleolus and associated with swelling; may be complaint of decreased range of motion (ROM) (see 13.1).

Si:
- Pt may have an antalgic gait or other gait abnormalities.
- Tenderness over the deltoid ligament, with or without edema or ecchymosis about the medial malleolus.
- Restricted active ROM.
- Assess posterior tibialis tendon (resisted eversion; see 13.7) and flexor hallucis longus (FHL; resisted flexion of great toe) function.
- Tibiofibular squeeze test for syndesmotic injury (see 13.4).
- Reverse talar tilt test for deltoid ligament stability (similar to talar tilt test, but with passive eversion of hind foot; see 13.1).
- Grading system similar to lateral sprains, but applied to deltoid ligament (see 13.1).
- Check for *maissoneurve* fracture (see 13.4).

Cmplc: Talar dome injuries (eg, OCD, see 13.5), syndesmotic injury (see 13.4), tib-fib fractures.

Diff Dx: Syndesmotic injury (see 13.4), posterior tibialis tendon injuries (see 13.7), talar dome injuries (see 13.5), ankle fracture, Achilles tendon rupture (see 13.6), midfoot injury (see 14.14), FHL injuries, tarsal coalition, sustentacular injury, tarsal tunnel syndrome.

X-ray: See X-ray section in 13.1.

Rx: See Rx section in 13.1.

13.3 Peroneal Tendon Subluxation and Dislocation

Handbook of Sports Medicine: A Symptom-Oriented Approach. 2nd ed. Boston: Butterworth and Heinemann 1999;287; Med Sci Sports Exerc 1999;31:S487

Cause: Acute dorsiflexion and inversion stress to the ankle.

Epidem: This injury is associated with a wide variety of sporting activity, most commonly in skiing (71%), football (7%), and basketball.

Pathophys: Sudden and forceful inversion and dorsiflexion of foot result in rupture of inferior or superior retinaculum, which normally channel the peroneal tendon, allowing peroneus brevis tendon to sublux anteriorly over posterior ridge of fibula; often occurs in conjunction with anterolateral ankle instability.

Sx: The athlete generally notes a "pop" and/or snapping sensation posterior to the lateral malleolus; pain or swelling may also be localized to this area.

Si: Tenderness and swelling posterior and inferior to lateral malleolus; palpable subluxation of the tendon or pain with active dorsiflexion and eversion against resistance.

Cmplc: Often misdiagnosed as lateral sprain; nonoperative treatment may lead to chronic lateral ankle pain and instability.

Diff Dx: More posterior peroneus longus tendon snapping over the more anterior peroneus brevis tendon; ankle sprain; fibular fracture.

X-ray: Radiographs may reveal a fracture-avulsion of the lateral ridge of the fibula.

Rx:
- Treatment in the active individual is controversial.
- Results with closed treatment are generally disappointing (recurrence rates of 50-70%).
- Consider early referral to orthopedics for surgical evaluation.

13.4 Syndesmosis Injury (High Ankle Sprain)

Phy Sportsmed 1993;21:39; J Am Acad Orthop Surg 1997;5:172; Clin Podiatr Med Surg 2001;18:443

Cause: Ankle pronation with abduction or external or internal rotation.

Epidem: Football, wrestling, and downhill skiing; ~1% of all ankle sprains.

Pathophs: Sudden, forceful abduction, internal rotation, external rotation, or extreme dorsiflexion forces the talus against the fibula,
opening the distal tibiofibular joint, and causing injury to the
syndesmotic ligaments of the ankle; the syndesmotic ligaments
consist of the anterior inferior tibiofibular ligament (AITFL), the
posterior inferior tibiofibular ligament (PITFL) and the interosseus ligament (IOM) (primary bond between the tibia and
fibula); can result in diastasis between the tibia and fibula at the
ankle.

Sx: Can appear benign initially; pain along the interosseus membrane,
pain proximal and anterior on the ankle; isolated injury to the
syndesmosis without fracture not common, and often associated
with medial ankle sprain; athlete presents with marked discomfort and swelling: often unable to bear wt.

Si:

- Often there is minimal swelling, especially in isolated injuries.
- There may be joint line tenderness at the anterior aspect of the
  ankle.
- Evaluate neurovascular status.
- Positive squeeze test:
  - Apply compression with one or two hands to the midpoint
    of the calf; the test is pos, if compression produces pain at
    distal tib-fib.
- Positive cotton test (or external rotation test):
  - Stabilize the distal lower leg with one hand while grasping
    each side of the foot at the tales with the thumb and forefin-
    ger of the other hand (Figure 13.2).
  - Apply a mediolateral force (externally rotate the foot) and
    assess crepitus, instability, or pain.
  - Increased motion or pain in the anterior tib-fib area or any-
    where along the fibula is a pos test.

Cmplc: Maissoneurve fracture, syndesmosis sprain with fracture, typically involves complete rupture of the deltoid ligament, the

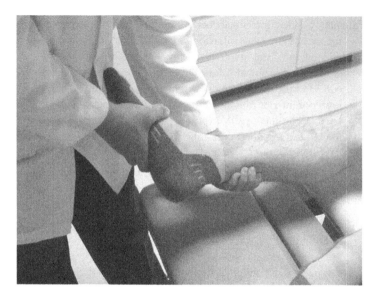

Figure 13.2 Cotton or external rotation test

ATFL, and IOM and a proximal fibula fracture; failure to recognize radiographic evidence of syndesmosis injury results in prolonged disability; bony avulsions from tibia; compartment syndrome; heterotopic ossification.

Diff Dx: Ankle sprain (see 13.1), OCD of the talar dome (see 13.5), loose body, instability, distal tib-fib fracture.

X-ray: Mortise view to assess mortise alignment of tibia, talus, and fibula; weight-bearing views recommended.
- Mortise view abnormal if:
  - The tibiofibular clear space is > 6 mm on AP and mortise views.
  - There is < 6 mm of overlap of the tibia and fibula at the fibularis incisura on AP view.

- Less than 1 mm of tibia and fibula overlap on the mortise view.
- Any difference of more than 5° between left and right talocrural angles (normal is 8-15°)
- Use comparison with uninjured ankle if unclear; AP and lateral of lower leg to rule out maissoneurve fracture.

Rx:

- For ankle sprain without fracture and without radiographic evidence of syndesmotic injury, standard ankle rehabilitation; recovery time 9 wk+.
- For injuries with radiographic evidence of syndesmotic injury, with or without associated fracture, refer to orthopedic surgeon for stabilization with syndesmosis screw.

13.5 Osteochondral Defect of the Talus (OCD)

Phy Sportsmed 1993;21:109; J Am Acad Orthop Sug 1996;4:63; J Bone Joint Surg 1959;41A:988

Cause: Traumatic or idiopathic etiologies.

Epidem: Osteochondral injuries/fractures commonly occur in association with inversion ankle sprains; OCL (osteochondral lesions) typically appear in the younger athlete.

Pathophys: These tibio-talar intra-articular fractures occur when there is a compressive component involved in the mechanism of injury; the fractures most commonly involve the anterolateral and posteromedial aspects of the talus; forceful inversion of the dorsi-flexed ankle impacts the talus onto the fibula, resulting in an intra-articular anterolateral lesion; posteromedial lesions result from inversion of the plantar-flexed ankle, impacting the talus onto the tibia.

Sx:

- Athlete describes vague pain "inside" his or her ankle.

- These injuries are frequently missed on initial examination and it is only when the pt presents with prolonged pain or aching, persistent swelling and/or perhaps catching, locking, or giving way that the diagnosis is contemplated.
- Activity-related swelling or pain, especially with wt-bearing activity.

Si:

- The pt may have tenderness over the dome of the talus.
- Tenderness to palpation over anterolateral or posteromedial aspect of ankle.
- Palpable lesion, detectable with posterior lesion in maximum plantar flexion, effusion, decreased range of motion, pain with inversion or eversion, and crepitus may be present.
- Exam may be normal.

Cmplc: Chronic ankle pain, accelerated OA, mechanical symptoms (locking) from loose body.

Diff Dx: Osteoarthritis, anterolateral soft tissue impingement (see 13.8), instability, poorly rehabilitated lateral ankle sprain (see 13.1), crystal-induced arthropathies.

X-ray:

- Findings often subtle; radiographs (plantar flexion views) may demonstrate a discrete fragment in an acute injury and subchondral sclerosis, and/or cysts in the subacute or chronic presentation.
- If plain films are normal, and the diagnostic suspicion is high, a bone scan with coned down views of foot and ankle should be ordered.
- Positive bone scan or plain films warrant further evaluation with a high resolution CT or MRI for staging.
- Berndt and Hardy Classification (J Bone Joint Surg 1959;41A:988):
  Stage I: Small area of compression.
  Stage II: Partially detached OCL.

Stage III: Completely detached, nondisplaced fragment.

Stage IV: Completely detached, displaced fragment; free body.

Rx: Refer for appropriate staging and management; treatment may range from a non-wt-bearing cast to open reduction and internal fixation.

13.6 Achilles Tendon Rupture

Am J Sports Med 1993;21:791; Clin J Sp Med 1997;7:207

Cause: Occurs after a sudden dorsiflexion of a plantar flexed foot; eccentric load from a cutting motion or sudden change of direction on a court.

Epidem: Commonly seen in athletes in the 4th and 5th decades of life; common in basketball, baserunning in baseball, or court sports; more commonly occurs in left Achilles tendon than right.

Pathophs: Rupture or partial rupture of Achilles tendon, usually between 2-6 cm proximal to calcaneal insertion: relative avascular zone 2-6 cm proximal to insertion.

Sx: The athlete may complain of a sudden "pop" in the heel or reports a feeling of being shot or kicked in the heel, followed by difficulty walking and pain with wt-bearing.

Si:

- May have a tender, palpable defect in the tendon 2-3 cm proximal to the heel (aka, "Hatchet strike" defect or sign).
- Positive Thompson test (Figure 13.3):
  - Pt lies prone on the examining table with the feet extending over the end of the exam table.
  - The examiner squeezes the middle third of the gastroc-soleus and observes for movement of the dorsiflexed foot into a position of plantar flexion.

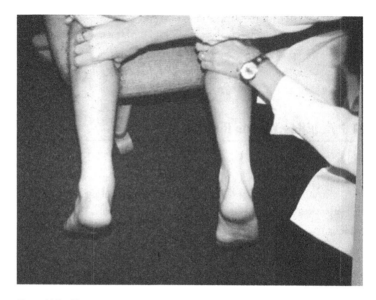

Figure 13.3 Thompson squeeze test

- The test can also be performed with the pt kneeling on a chair.
- Absence of plantar flexion suggests a disruption of the Achilles tendon.

Cmplc: Failure to promptly diagnose may limit operative repair and prolong disability; ankle sprain is the most common initial misdiagnosis.

Diff Dx: Gastroc or soleus strain (see 12.3), Achilles tendinopathy (see 13.12), retrocalcaneal bursitis (see 14.17); Achilles bursitis, calcaneal avulsion fracture, ankle sprain.

X-ray: If necessary MRI can establish a definitive diagnosis; plain films may be helpful in excluding a calcaneal avulsion fracture.

Rx:

- Initial management: posterior, non-wt-bearing splint with 45° plantar flexion; crutches, ice, pain medications, elevation.
- Refer for operative repair, which has been demonstrated to provide superior strength, endurance, and a lower risk of re-rupture in the athlete.
- Nonoperative treatment usually recommended for less active, elderly pts, or those with contraindications to surgery.
- If nonoperative treatment is elected, cast in gravity equinus position (gravity induced plantar flexion) in long or short leg cast; no wt-bearing on leg for 8 wk, crutches for mobility; consider recasting in reduced plantar flexion at 4 wk; after 8 wk, the cast is removed and a 2.5-cm heel lift is worn for 4 wk.
- Rehabilitation with passive, then active range-of-motion and strengthening exercises, including heel raises; proprioceptive rehabilitation is also important.
- There is an increased risk of deep vein thrombosis (DVT) with prolonged casting: consider anticoagulation for DVT prophylaxis in high-risk pts.

13.7 Posterior Tibialis Tendon Rupture

Handbook of Sports Medicine: A Symptom-Oriented Approach. 2nd ed. Boston: Butterworth and Heinemann 1999;283; Clin Podiatr Med Surg 2000;17:33

Cause: Sudden plantar flexion, usually preceded by chronic medial ankle pain and associated with aging.

Epidem: Common clinical entity seen in mature female athletes who engage in hiking and patients with hypermobile flat feet; also seen in sports requiring quick changes in direction (eg, soccer and basketball); most common cause of acquired flatfoot deformity.

Pathophys: The repetitive microtrauma of excessive pronation is thought to result in degenerative changes in tendon leading to acute disruption.

Sx: Difficulty walking with or without pain and swelling immediately posterior to the medial malleolus; pain is worse with ambulation; rarely associated with trauma.

Si:

- Classically the pt presents with *unilateral fallen arch* when standing *(pes planus)*.
- When viewed from behind, the pt demonstrates the "too many toes" sign on the lateral aspect of the affected foot secondary to abduction of the forefoot *(pes valgus)*.
- When the pt is asked to stand on his toes, the affected foot is unable to demonstrate the normal inversion secondary to an absent posterior tibialis.
- Soft tissue swelling posterior to the medial malleolus; the pain is aggravated by inversion and plantar flexion against resistance.

Cmplc: Potential for severe disability.

X-ray: In cases where the diagnosis is unclear, MRI is the test of choice.

Rx: Refer for operative repair, and/or tendon transfers, in cases of rupture.

Chronic Injuries

13.8 Anterolateral and Syndesmotic Soft Tissue Impingement

Am J Sports Med 1998;253:89; Foot Ankle Int 2004;25:63

Cause: Anterolateral impingement of the ankle soft tissues secondary to repeated ankle sprains.

Epidem: Activities such as gymnastics, tennis, basketball, volleyball, soccer, football, and ballet have been commonly noted to result in anterior tibiotalar impingement; often seen in athlete whose ankle is not aggressively rehabilitated after previous sprain.

Pathophys: The dome of the talus rubs against a hypertrophied and scarred anterior inferior tibiofibular ligament (AITFL) or anterior talofibular ligament (ATFL), causing reactive tissue formation; repeated injury can result in synovial hypertrophy and/or a meniscoid lesion that is commonly identified in the anterolateral gutter.

Sx: Chronic, persistent, vague anterior ankle pain, intermittent catching, and/or swelling; generally worse with activity; occasionally, a "popping" or "snapping" sensation with dorsiflexion; pain with walking uphill.

Si: The most ratable clinical finding is restriction and painful dorsiflexion of the ankle; tenderness to palpation over the anterior talocrural joint, lateral gutter, ATFL; in syndesmotic impingement, may have pain with bimalleolar compression.

Cmplc: Progression to constant pain.

Diff Dx: Loose body, OCD (see 13.5), OA, peroneal tendon tendinopathy or subluxation (see 13.3), tarsal coalition, tarsal tunnel syndrome (see 14.18), RSD/CRPS.

X-ray: Exostoses are generally present on lateral radiographs; oblique radiographs may also be helpful; non-wt-bearing lateral flexion and extension views will demonstrate the impingement; plain films, bone scan, and CT scans may be normal.

Rx:
- Aggressive Achilles stretching program, relative rest, and modification of activity (eg, no hill running).
- Ice and contrast baths to affected area.
- Diagnosis may be confirmed with single injection of the ATFL with 1 cc lidocaine.

- If pos, good response to diagnostic injection, the provider may consider a follow-up injection with lidocaine and 6 mg celestone or 20 mg kenalog for treatment (see 1.14).
- Failure of 4 wks of conservative therapy should be referred for possible arthroscopic debridement or resection.

13.9 Posterior Tibialis Tendinopathy

The Lower Extremity and Spine in Sports Medicine. 2nd ed. St. Louis: Mosby 1995;441; Clin Podiatr Med Surg 2000;17:33

Cause: Degenerative changes in tendon associated with aging.

Epidem: Common clinical entity seen in mature female athletes who engage in hiking and pts with hypermobile flat feet; also seen in sports requiring quick changes in direction (eg, soccer and basketball).

Pathophys: The repetitive microtrauma of excessive pronation is thought to result in degenerative changes in tendon leading to acute disruption.

Sx: Difficulty walking; pain and swelling immediately posterior to the medial malleolus; the pain is worse when bearing weight and ambulating; rarely associated with trauma.

Si: Tenderness to palpation immediately posterior to the medial malleolus, frequently associated crepitance; soft tissue swelling posterior to the medial malleolus; the pain is aggravated by inversion and plantar flexion against resistance.

Cmplc: Rupture, tarsal tunnel syndrome, chronic pain, and dysfunction.

Diff Dx: Tarsal tunnel syndrome (see 14.18), tarsal navicular stress fracture (see 14.11), deltoid ligament sprain.

X-ray: MRI may demonstrate degeneration.

Rx:

- Rest, modification of abusive activities (including wt-bearing, if aggravating).
- Ice, massage.
- NSAIDs
- Foot orthosis to decrease pronation.
- Physical therapy for Achilles stretching, resistive posterior tibialis strengthening.
- Slow toe raises, accentuating the lowering phase, should be started when able to do the exercise pain free.
- In the young athlete with acute inflammation or in severe cases, immobilization in a short leg, non-wt-bearing cast with the foot in slight inversion for 10 d often relieves the symptoms.
- Refer refractory cases to consider surgical management (tenodesis or tendon transfer augmentation)

13.10 Sinus Tarsi Syndrome

The Lower Extremity and Spine in Sports Medicine. 2nd ed. St. Louis: Mosby 1995;437; Phy Sportsmed 2000;28:75

Cause: Posttraumatic, forceful inversion of the foot.

Epidem: History of multiple prior ankle sprains.

Pathophys: The syndrome is generally secondary to a prolonged synovitis following an injury to the subtalar ligaments; one proposed factor in the pathogenesis is posttraumatic fibrotic changes in the tissue surrounding the veins draining the sinus, resulting in increased intrasinusal pressure (Clin Anat 1997;10:173).

Sx: Pain over the lateral opening of the sinus tarsi (talocalcaneal sulcus) along with a feeling of instability; pain while walking on uneven surfaces or down steps.

Si: Tenderness over lateral side of the foot that is increased by firm pressure over the sinus tarsi and inversion of the foot, but ameliorated by eversion of the foot; relief with 2-3 cc of lidocaine directly into the sinus tarsi confirms the diagnosis; ankle is otherwise stable.

Cmplc: Chronic pain.

Diff Dx: Anterolateral soft tissue impingement (see 14.8), lateral ankle sprain (see 13.1), bifurcate ligament injury, cuboid/talus/calcaneal stress fracture (see 14.13), OA, OCD (see 13.5).

X-ray: Radiographs are unremarkable; MRI may be considered if diagnosis unclear or for surgical planning.

Rx: Treatment is difficult and should include complete ankle rehabilitation; relative rest, avoidance of aggravating activities, orthotics if indicated, and NSAIDs should be started; if unsuccessful, corticosteroid injection to the sinus tarsi may provide relief: multiple injections may be necessary; if conservative treatment fails, surgical debridement of the sinus tarsi can be helpful.

13.11 Distal Fibular Stress Fracture

Handbook of Sports Medicine: A Symptom-Oriented Approach. 2nd ed. Boston: Butterworth and Heinemann 1999;27

Cause: History of overuse and activity-related lateral ankle pain.

Epidem: Runners, military recruits.

Pathophs: Chronic insult to distal fibula gradually fatigues and eventually leads to cortical failure, faster than bone remodeling can prevent the break.

Sx: On occasion the athlete may note some mild swelling above the lateral ankle; the pain generally improves with rest; symptoms usually gradual in onset over a 2-3-wk period.

Si: Focal bony tenderness 2-7 cm proximal to the lateral malleolus.

Cmplc: Complete fracture, may become displaced.

Diff Dx: Peroneal tendinopathy or strain (see 13.3), exertional compartment syndrome (see 12.2).

X-ray: Radiographs frequently reveal a focal periosteal reaction; if neg, a bone scan is confirmatory.

Rx: Stop abusive activity for a period of 4-6 wk as the bone remodels; the athlete may participate in non-wt-bearing cross training activities; upon return to sport, shock absorbing insoles and "forgiving" running surfaces may help; the most important preventive feature, however, is to avoid doing too much, too soon.

13.12 Achilles Tendinopathy

Am J Sports Med 1998;26:360

Cause: Overuse, increase in mileage, increase in hill running, poor calf/hamstring flexibility.

Epidem: Common injury in runners and athletes 30-40 y/o.

Pathophys:
- Degenerative changes in Achilles tendon from chronic insult.
- Histology of affected tendons reveal this condition (and other chronic overuse injuries) is not associated with inflammation, hence the term tendinopathy rather than familiar tendinitis, which implies inflammation.

Sx: Activity-related pain localized to the tendon, approximately 3-4 cm above its insertion into the calcaneus; recent change in shoes and/or training; morning stiffness.

Si: Tenderness and possibly focal swelling and/or crepitus in the tendon; in chronic tendinopathy the tendon is often thickened and nodular; hamstring and gastroc-soleus inflexibility, as well as evidence of functional overpronation are common; normal Thompson test (see 13.6, Fig. 13.3).

Cmplc: Achilles tendon rupture (see 14.6), chronic pain, and dysfunction.

Diff Dx: Peritendonitis, retrocalcaneal bursitis (see 14.17).

X-ray: MRI of lower leg if confirmation is needed.

Rx:

Initial: Relative rest from the offending activity (cross train); then modification of activities to include decreasing mileage and avoiding hill-running; orthotics to correct pathologic over-pronation; heavy eccentric (stretching phase) exercise:

- The patient raises one toe using the healthy leg and lowers to the ground using the injured leg for 15 reps and 3 sets with the injured leg straight and 15 reps with the injured flexed 15°.
- Additional wt is added in a backpack as strength is gained.
- Gentle slow calf stretching on slant board or block is performed at least 3 × d.
- This routine is done daily for 3 mo with gradual return to running as tolerated during this time.

Severe cases: Can be temporarily casted in the equines (plantar flexed) position for 2-4 wk; refer recalcitrant cases for surgical debridement (although many surgeons recommend consistent physical therapy and/or rehabilitation for 3 mo before considering surgery).

Chapter 14

The Foot

Skin and Nails

14.1 Blisters

Phy Sportsmed 2004;32:36; Curr Sports Med Rep 2002;1:319

Cause: Repeated friction on the skin surface.

Epidem: Common, potentially debilitating injury; often occur early in the season.

Pathophys: Acute response to high-intensity stress, which produces a shear force which separates the skin into 2 layers; the space fills w fluid secondary to hemodynamic forces.

Sx: Pain.

Si: Vessicle, which may be filled w blood or purulent fluid; tender to palpation.

Crs: May rupture w persistent activity.

Cmplc: May become infected.

Rx:
- Prevention includes appropriately fitted shoes and socks, padding hot spots, lubricants.
- Acute treatment includes possible drainage, use of a blister care product (second skin, sports patch, etc.), antibiotic ointment, and protective padding.
- Care must be taken to keep the site clean to avoid infection.

14.2 Subungal Hematoma

Am Fam Phys 2005;71:856; J Am Acad Dermatol 2003;48:58

Cause: Improperly fitted shoes; downhill running; direct trauma.

Epidem: Common in long-distance runners.

Pathophys: Shearing or crushing injury in which there is bleeding under the toenail.

Sx: Pain.

Si: Blood under the nail; may be tender.

Crs: Gradually resolves. The nail may fall off at some future point.

Cmplc: Loss of the nail; subsequent nail abnormality.

X-ray: Rule out fracture in cases of direct trauma.

Rx:

- Appropriately fitted shoes may prevent this problem.
- If hemorrhage is acute and painful, it can be relieved by drilling a hole in the nail, using a heated 18-g needle or the end of an opened paperclip or a battery-operated cautery (beware of converting a closed fx to an open fx).
- A sterile dressing should be applied.

Forefoot Problems

14.3 Hallux Valgus

DeLee and Drez's Orthopaedic Sports Medicine. Philadelphia: WB Saunders 2003;2483; Textbook of Running Medicine. New York: McGraw-Hill 2001;218

Cause: Previous injury; congenital factors.

Epidem: Congenital and familial factors; previous injury, ie, first MTP dislocation, turf toe, rupture of the joint capsule; overpronation.

Pathophys: Lateral deviation of the proximal phalanx on the first metatarsal; the medial aspect of the head of the first metatarsal enlarges and the overlying bursa becomes inflamed and thickened (bunion).

Sx: Pain; deformity.

Si: Deformity of the first MTP joint; may be tender to palpation.

Crs: Valgus deformity may progress.

Cmplc: Degenerative changes in the MTP joint and hallux limitus or rigidus may develop (see 15.9).

X-ray: Valgus deformity of first MTP joint; degenerative joint disease.

Rx:
- Shoes with a wide toe box; padding around the metatarsal prominence.
- Orthotic devices if overpronation or Morton's toe are present.
- Surgery for persistent pain despite conservative management.

14.4 Turf Toe

DeLee and Drez's Orthopaedic Sports Medicine. Philadelphia: WB Saunders 2003;2504; Clin Sports Med 2004;23:115

Cause: Hyperextension of the first MTP joint.

Epidem: Flexible shoes and faster playing surfaces increase the incidence of this injury.

Pathophys: Injury to the capsuloligamentous complex of the first MTP joint secondary to hyperextension of the joint.

Sx: Pain, especially w ambulation.

Si: Pain w passive extension of the first MTP joint; swelling and ecchymosis may be present.
Grade 1: pain in plantar and medial aspect of MTP joint, minimal swelling.

Grade 2: increased pain swelling and ecchymosis.

Grade 3: severe pain, marked swelling and ecchymosis.

Crs: Gradual improvement w treatment.

Cmplc: Persistent pain; joint instability.

Diff Dx: Gout, MTP OA (see 14.9), Sesmoiditis (see 14.10).

X-ray: Usually neg; small avulsion fracture may be present.

Rx:

Rest, ice, elevation, NSAIDs:

Grade 1: shoe w stiff sole or orthoses with Morton's extension; taping.

Grade 2: same as grade 1; return to activity when sxs diminish (1-2 wks).

Grade 3: crutches for several d; orthoses with Morton's extension; physical therapy modalities; return to activity in 3-6 wks; if sxs of persistent pain, joint instability and swelling, surgery may be required.

14.5 Hallux Rigidus

Clin Sports Med 2000;19:33; Textbook of Running Medicine. New York: McGraw-Hill 2001;217

Cause: Degenerative changes of the first MTP joint.

Epidem: Congenital abnormalities; osteochondritis of the metatarsal head; overpronation; trauma.

Pathophys: Painful restricted motion of the first MTP joint secondary to degenerative changes.

Sx: Pain with walking or running.

Si: Pain and swelling of the first MTP joint; restricted extension; pain w forced extension; palpable bony ridge along the dorsal aspect of the joint.

Crs: Pain w activity may increase as degenerative changes progress.

Cmplc: Tendonitis, plantar fasciitis (see 15.19) or other injury secondary to compensation for altered gait.

Diff Dx: Turf toe (see 14.8), sesmoiditis (see 14.10).

X-ray: Bony exostoses and degenerative joint disease.

Rx:
- Shoes with wide toe box and rigid sole.
- NSAIDs.
- Rocker bottom shoe.
- Surgery.

14.6 Sesamoid Problems

Clin Sports Med 2000;19:34; DeLee and Drez's Orthopaedic Sports Medicine. Philadelphia: WB Saunders 2003;2510

Cause: Acute or overuse injury.

Epidem: Repetitive stress or landing on the first MTP joint; increased incidence w pes cavus.

Pathophys: Inflammation or fracture of one of the sesamoids:
- Sesamoiditis: tendonitis, bursitis, or chrondromalacia.
- Sesamoid stress fracture: similar to sesamoiditis, w persistent pain despite conservative management; pos bone scan.
- Acute fracture: usually a transverse compression fracture of the medial sesamoid caused by landing on the ball of the foot.

Sx: Acute or insidious onset of pain; pain w toe-off.

Si: Pain on palpation of one of the sesamoids (typically medial); swelling may be present; painful and possibly restricted extension of the great toe.

Crs: Persistent or worsening symptoms without treatment; often requires prolonged course of treatment.

Cmplc: Persistent pain despite treatment; nonunion of fracture.

Diff Dx: Tendonitis, 1st MTP OA (see 14.9)

X-ray: (Sesamoid view) May demonstrate an acute fracture or stress
fracture which has been present for several wks. Bone scan or CT
is useful if plain radiographs are neg, but sxs are suggestive of an
acute or stress fracture.

Rx:
- Sesamoiditis:
  - Ice.
  - NSAIDs.
  - Padding to unload the first metatarsal head.
  - Semi-rigid orthoses.
- Sesamoid stress fracture:
  - Short leg walking cast for 6 wk.
  - Use of orthoses to unload the metatarsal head upon return to
    sports; acute sesamoid fracture: short leg walking cast for
    6 wk or taping toe in neutral position, w padding proximal
    to the sesamoids and use of a wooden soles postoperative
    shoe. If there is nonunion of a fracture, and/or persistent
    pain, surgical excision or partial excision may be necessary.

14.7 Morton's Neuroma

Med Clin N Amer 2003;87:690; Am Fam Phys 2003;68:1360

Cause: Repetitive microtrauma.

Epidem: Trauma occurs during toe off phase of running or w repetitive
episodes of rising on toes; most commonly between the third and
fourth metatarsal heads.

Pathophys: Repetitive microtrauma of the interdigital nerve at the
distal edge of the intermetatarsal ligament in the narrow intermetatarsal space causes perineural fibrosis; the nerve is stressed as
the third metatarsal extends more than the fourth metatarsal.

Sx: Complaint of plantar or forefoot burning, cramping, or pain; numbness in toes

Si: Tenderness with squeezing the web space (most commonly the third web space, occasionally the second). A palpable clicking may be noted when the thumb is rolled distally into the interspace from the metatarsal head level on the plantar aspect; movement of the neuroma over the intermetatarsal ligament produces a painful click (Mulder's sign).

Cmplc: Chronic pain and dysestheias.

Diff Dx: Metatarsal stress fracture (see 14.15), Freiberg's infarction (see 14.8).

X-ray: Unremarkable.

Rx: Shoes w wide toe box; metatarsal pad in the affected web space; NSAIDs; one or two steroid injections; if symptoms persist, surgery.

14.8 Freiberg's Infarction

DeLee and Drez's Orthopaedic Sports Medicine. Philadelphia: WB Saunders 2003;2387; Prim Care 2005;32:105; Prim Care 2005;32:133

Cause: Repetitive microtrauma; hypermobile first metatarsal.

Epidem: Typical age at presentation is 13 yr; 75% are female.

Pathophys: Avascular necrosis of the second metatarsal epiphysis.

Sx: Pain w activities.

Si: Pain on palpation of head of second metatarsal (less commonly third, fourth, or fifth).

Crs: Usually self-limited.

Cmplc: Chronic pain, accelerated OA.

Diff Dx: Metatarsal stress fx (see 14.15), metatarsalgia, Morton's neuroma (see 14.11).

X-ray: Osteosclerosis progressing to osteolysis of the metatarsal head.

Rx: Orthoses; short leg cast for severe pain; physical therapy to restore joint motion; rarely needs surgery.

14.9 Phalangeal Fractures

Am Fam Phys 2003;68:2413; Ortho Clin North Am 2001;32:1

Cause: Trauma; jamming or stubbing.

Epidem: Uncommon in great toe.

Pathophys: Bone is unable to withstand the energy generated by trauma.

Sxs: History of trauma; pain; swelling.

Si: Pain, swelling, deformity, ecchymosis.

Crs: Fracture healing.

Cmplc: Malunion or nonunion; open fracture.

X-ray: Confirm fracture.

Rx: Uncomplicated fracture: buddy taping w padding between toes; shoe with stiff sole and wide toe box.
- Refer: large intra-articular fracture; severely displaced fracture; open fracture.

14.10 Metatarsal Fracture

Ortho Clin North Am 2001;32:1; Clin Fam Practice 2000;2:661

Cause: Due to direct trauma or inversion/eversion of the forefoot.

Pathophys: Bone is unable to withstand the energy generated either directly or indirectly.

Sx: History of trauma; pain; swelling.

Si: Localized tenderness, swelling, crepitus, ecchymosis.

Crs: Fracture healing.

Cmplc: Malunion or nonunion; open fracture.

Diff Dx: Lisfranc joint injury (see 14.18), tendonitis, midfoot OA.

X-ray: Direct trauma produces transverse or short oblique fracture.
   • Indirect trauma produces spiral fracture.

Rx: Comfort and protection: cast, postop shoe, strapping. Multiple fractures: short leg walking cast.
   Refer:
   • First metatarsal fractures (significant wt-bearing role).
   • Displaced fractures (bone ends have shifted relative to one another).
   • Fractures at base of metatarsals (beware of Lisfranc fracture dislocation).

14.11 Metatarsal Stress Fracture

Clin J Sp Med 2003;13:358; Am Fam Phys 2003;68:1527

Cause: Recurrent microtrauma.

Epidem: Common in running and jumping sports.

Pathophys: Secondary repetitive activities (running, aerobics, etc). Often associated w increased training. Other contributing factors include inadequate shoes, training surface, biomechanical abnormalities, and osteopenia. Most commonly occur in second metatarsal, followed by the third metatarsal. The first metatarsal is the most mobile and the second is the most stable, making the latter susceptible to stress.

Sx: Aching or pain in the forefoot w activity, often associated w a sudden increase in training.

Si: Localized tenderness on palpation of metatarsal.

Cmplc: Complete fracture.

Diff Dx: Tendonitis.

X-ray: Initially normal; after 2 wk: periosteal reaction, callus formation, cortical thickening, cortical interruption may be seen.

Rx:

- Minimal discomfort: limitation of wt-bearing activity; post-op shoe or strapping; non-wt-bearing cross training (swimming, cycling, pool running, etc); determine and correct cause of injury; gradual return to activities.
- Severe pain: short leg walking cast for 4-6 wk.

14.12 Fifth Metatarsal Fracture

Ortho Clin North Am 2001;32:171; Clin J Sp Med 2003;13:358

1. Acute Fracture Without Evidence of Preexisting Injury (History of Pain or Changes on Radiographs)

Cause: Direct trauma or inversion injury.

Epidem: Fairly common injury.

Pathophys:
- Inversion injury of forefoot: spiral fracture of shaft.
- Inversion injury of ankle: avulsion fracture of base of metatarsal.

Sx: History of trauma; pain.

Si: Localized tenderness, swelling, ecchymosis, crepitus.

Crs: Healing fracture.

Cmplc: Malunion or nonunion; open fracture.

X-ray: Clean fracture line; avulsion fracture is at right angle to shaft of metatarsal (apophysis seen in 8-12 y/o is longitudinally oriented).

Rx:
- Fracture of shaft: short leg walking cast or boot for 4-6 wk; displaced fracture should be referred.
- Avulsion fracture: strapping and post-op shoe.

2. Fracture With Evidence of Preexisting Injury

Cause: Repetitive microtrauma.

Epidem: Often complain of pain prior to acute injury.

Pathophys: Repetitive microtrauma (see metatarsal stress fracture). Jones fracture is a stress fracture of the proximal diaphysis of the fifth metatarsal.

Sx: Pain in the proximal fifth metatarsal with wt-bearing activities; may complain of a pop or sudden onset of severe pain.

Si: Localized tenderness on palpation.

Cmplc: High incidence of delayed union or nonunion.

X-ray: Transverse proximal diaphyseal fracture; look for preexisting stress reaction: radiolucent fracture line, periosteal reaction, callus formation with sclerosis.

Rx:
- Discuss all cases with orthopedic surgeon.
- Non-wt-bearing cast for 4-6 wk, followed by 4+ wk in wt-bearing cast.
- May require surgical fixation.

Midfoot Problems

14.13 Tarsal Navicular Stress Fracture

Phy Sportsmed 2005;33:28; Am Fam Phys 2003;67:85

Cause: Repetitive microtrauma.

Epidem: Seen in distance runners and jumpers.

Pathophys: Repetitive microtrauma (see 14.11)

Sx: Vague pain in dorsal, medial aspect of midfoot aggravated by activity.

Si: Tenderness on palpation of navicular, usually without swelling.

Cmplc: High incidence of delayed union and nonunion.

Diff Dx: Tendonitis, OA.

X-ray: Often normal; may see sclerotic line in navicular; bone scan will be pos; tomograms or CT will demonstrate vertical fracture.

Rx:

- Poor blood supply to navicular and high frequency of delayed union and nonunion make this a difficult fracture to treat.
- Discuss all cases with orthopedic surgeon.
- Displaced fractures should be referred.
- Non-wt-bearing cast for 6-8 wk; resume full activity in 3-6 mo.

14.14 Lisfranc Fracture-Dislocation

Clin Sports Med 2004;23:105; Am J EM 2001;19:71

Cause: Direct or indirect trauma.

Epidem: Uncommon injury in sports.

Pathophys: The Lisfranc joint is the tarsal-metatarsal joints. Includes articulation of bases of five metatarsals with three cuneiforms and cuboid. Second metatarsal is key stabilizer of this joint; even minor subluxation of this joint can de-stabilize the entire forefoot.

- Direct trauma: foot run over by a vehicle; heavy wt dropped on foot.
- Indirect trauma: hyperplantar flexion of forefoot w dorsal displacement of proximal ends of metatarsals; fall on pointed toes; fall backward while forefoot is trapped; sudden high-velocity longitudinal compression.

Sx: Pain often seems exaggerated. Unable to bear wt.

Si: Pain and swelling of dorsum of foot; soft tissue damage w direct trauma; neurovascular exam very important due to potential compartment syndrome in foot.

Cmplc: Permanent pain and disability.

Diff Dx: Tarsal or metatarsal fx (see 14.14, 14.17), midfoot OA.

X-ray: Often see small avulsion fracture at base of first or second metatarsal; spontaneous reduction is not uncommon; look for subtle malalignments on (wt-bearing) radiographs.

Normal AP: first metatarsal aligns w first cuneiform laterally and medially; medial border of second metatarsal aligns w medial border of second cuneiform.

Oblique: lateral border of third metatarsal aligns w lateral border of third cuneiform and medial border of fourth metatarsal aligns w medial border of cuboid.

Lateral: look for dorsal displacement of base of second metatarsal.

Rx:
- Recognition of this injury is essential.
- It is easy to incorrectly refer to orthopedics due to high incidence of complications.

Hindfoot Problems

14.15 Plantar Fasciitis

Clin J Sp Med 2004;14:305; Am Fam Phys 2001;63:477; Clin Sports Med 2004;23:123

Cause: Cavus foot, hyperpronation, excessive training, tight Achilles (heel cord).

Epidem: Most common cause of heel pain.

Pathophys: Traction periostitis at origin of plantar fascia at medial tuberosity of anterior calcaneus w subsequent degeneration and tears.

Sx: Insidious onset of heel pain. "First step pain" or pain w first few steps in morning or after long rest and pain after prolonged activity.

Si: Point tenderness medial tubercle of calcaneus; may also be tender along the longitudinal arch.

Crs: Tends to get worse over time.

Cmplc: Rupture of plantar fascia.

Diff Dx: Calcaneal stress fracture (see 14.20), neuroma (lateral plantar nerve), tarsal tunnel syndrome (see 14.22).

X-ray: Calcaneal plantar enthesiophyte may be seen.

Rx:

Initially:
- NSAIDs.
- Heel cord stretching.
- Cross friction massage (massage against the grain).
- Ice.
- Physical therapy modalities.
- Arch supports/heel cups/arch taping.
- Counterforce bracing.
- No barefoot walking.
- Limit wt-bearing activities—no running or jumping while symptomatic.
- Cross train in pool or on bicycle.

If symptoms persist:
- Night splints.
- Possible cortisone injections (see 2.16).
- Short leg walking cast for resistant cases.
- Occasionally, surgery is needed for persistent symptoms.

14.16 Calcaneal Stress Fracture

Am Fam Phys 2004;70:332; Clin Sports Med 2004;23:69

Cause: Maybe related to a sudden increase in activity.

Epidem: Usually related to sudden increase in activities.

Pathophys: Repetitive microtrauma (see 14.11)

Sx: Insidious onset of heel pain.

Si: Pain in posterior heel, especially w medial-lateral compression.

Crs: Progressive pain.

Cmplc: Complete fracture is not common.

Diff Dx: Plantar fasciitis (see 14.19), neuroma, tarsal tunnel syndrome (see 14.22).

X-ray: Normal in the first two wks; afterwards may demonstrate a trabecular linear density; bone scan will be pos in 48 hr.

Rx: Crutches or cast until asymptomatic, then padding (ice, heel cups); non-wt-bearing cross training; gradual return to activities.

14.17 Retrocalcaneal Bursitis

Am Fam Phys 2004;70:332

Cause: Rapid increase in activities; poorly fitting shoes.

Epidem: May be seen in pts with gout.

Pathophys: Inflammation of the retrocalcaneal bursa (between posterior calcaneus and anterior Achilles tendon) and the Achilles tendon insertion; there is often enlargement of the superior tuberosity of the os calcis.

Sx: Insidious onset of posterior heel pain, which is aggravated by increased activities and shoes w tight heel counter.

Si: Swelling between calcaneus and distal Achilles tendon; tenderness; prominent superior tuberosity of os calcis.

Crs: Increasing pain and swelling w persistent pressure.

Cmplc: Achilles tendonitis or rupture.

Diff Dx: Calcaneal stress fx (see 14.20), os trigonum injury (see 14.23), Achilles tendinopathy (see 13.15), tarsal tunnel syndrome (see 14.22).

THE FOOT

X-ray: May demonstrate Haglund's deformity (soft tissue changes of bursitis and tendonitis, plus a prominent bursal projection on the posterior calcaneus).

Rx:

- Appropriately fitted footwear may prevent the problem.
- Padding of posterior heel ("U" pad).
- Achilles tendon stretching.
- NSAIDs.
- Ice.
- Physical therapy modalities.

14.18 Tarsal Tunnel Syndrome

Med Clin N Amer 2003;87:684; Am Fam Phys 2003;68:1359

Cause: Nerve compression.

Epidem: Uncommon; improperly fitted shoes are a major factor.

Pathophys:

Tarsal Tunnel: The lacunate ligament makes up the roof and the plantar surfaces of the tarsal bones and the proximal metatarsals. The tunnel includes posterior tibial tendon, flexor digitorum longus tendon, and posterior tibial neurovascular bundle. After the posterior tibial nerve emerges from the tunnel, it splits into three branches: medial calcaneal sensory to the heel, medial plantar motor and sensory to the medial foot, and lateral plantar motor and sensory to the lateral foot. Compression of the posterior tibial nerve as it passes through the tarsal tunnel causes sxs. Contributing factors include joint instability, bony impingement (osteophyte, os rigonum, etc), space occupying lesion (ganglion cyst, venous varicosity, lipoma), and biomechanical abnormalities (overpronation). In 50% of cases, the cause is idiopathic.

Sx: Medial posterior foot pain, accompanied by burning and tingling; pain is exacerbated by standing and activity; may complain of night pain.

Si: Evaluate foot and ankle for swelling, presence of arches, bony prominences; percussion along the posterior tibial nerve may produce a pos Tinel's sign; there may be weakness of toe flexion and loss of two-point discrimination.

Crs: Progressive pain.

Cmplc: Weakness; loss of two-point discrimination.

Diff Dx: Calcaneal stress fx (see 14.20), radiculopathy (see 9.2), posterior tibialis tendinopathy (see 13.12).

Lab: EMG and NCV may be prolonged; these studies may be normal if compression is related to activity (ie, overpronation).

X-ray: May demonstrate osteophytes or an os trigonum.

Rx:
- NSAIDs.
- Correction of biomechanical abnormalities (arch support, medial wedge).
- Cortisone injection.
- Stretching.
- Cast immobilization.
- Surgical decompression if symptoms persist.

14.19 Os Trigonum Syndrome (Posterior Impingement)

Clin Sports Med 2000;19:30; Prim Care 2004;31:1055

Cause: Accessory ossicle posterior aspect of talus.

Epidem: Os trigonum is present in 10% of population; common problem in ballet, gymnastics, and jumping sports.

Pathophys: Excessive plantar flexion of ankle impinges the soft tissues on the bony process (os trigonum).

Sx: Pain with plantarflexion.

Si: Pain on palpation of posterior ankle, which increases significantly with forced plantarflexion.

Crs: Sxs occur with less activity.

Diff Dx: Acute fracture of os trigonum or posterior process of talus, retrocalcaneal bursitis (see 14.21).

X-ray: Ossicle is seen posterior to talus; en pointe view is helpful.

Rx:

- Ice.
- Activity modification.
- NSAIDs.
- Surgery may be necessary in recalcitrant cases (usually female dancers).

Chapter 15

Neurology

Headaches

15.1 Benign Exertional Headache

Clin Sports Med 1992;11:339

Cause: Excessive strain.

Epidem:
- Athletes are susceptible at the same rate as the general population for headaches of all kinds (muscle tension, vascular, posttraumatic, etc).
- In addition, there are several entities peculiar to certain athletes.

Pathophys: Due to decreased cerebral blood flow following exertion related increase in intracranial pressure via Valsalva effect.

Sx:
- Sudden onset, severe pain in a rapid crescendo pattern w dull headache.
- Usually occipital.
- Pain is worsened with continued effort.

Si: Generally nonspecific.

Crs: Symptoms last from a few min to several hr.

X-ray:
- CT or MRI recommended to rule out organic cause. Has been reported to be associated with structural lesion in up to 10% of cases.

Rx:
- NSAIDs.
- Biofeedback.
- Activity modification.

15.2 Weightlifter's Headache

Clin Sports Med 1992;11:339

Cause: Excessive straining.

Pathophys: Related to either increased intracranial pressure (Valsalva) or cervical ligament and tendon strain.

Sx: Sudden onset, severe and stabbing pain radiating from the base of the skull and proximal cervical spine to the parietal areas.

Si:
- Point tender at base of skull and posterior cervical structures.
- Painful ROM.
- Neurologic exam normal.

Crs: Variable.

X-ray:
- Cervical radiographs to rule out degenerative disease or structural anomaly.
- CT or MRI to rule out mass lesion, vascular lesion or Arnold-Chiari malformation.

Lab: Lumbar puncture to rule out infectious cause.

Rx:
- Analgesic measures: NSAIDS, cryotherapy, heat packs, analgesic medications, and massage.

- Physical therapy for scapulothoracic dysfunction, and cervical strengthening.

15.3 Exertional Migraine (Acute Effort Migraine)

Clin Sports Med 1992;11:339

Cause: Arise with brief, high-intensity effort.

Pathophys:
- Similar to migraine with hyperventilation leading to vasoconstriction (due to decreased pCO_2) followed by reflex vasodilation and headache.
- Contributing factors include: dehydration, exercising in extreme heat, poor nutrition, and alcohol consumption.

Sx:
- May have prodrome.
- Severe pain, short in duration.

Si: Negative exam.

Crs: Intense pain, short in duration.

Diff Dx: Other intense headache; intracranial mass, hemorrhage, infection, migraine.

X-ray: MRI indicated in general work-up of severe headache, but neg with acute effort migraine.

Rx:
- Treat as for typical migraine; NSAIDs, sumatriptan, ergotamine, or midrin.
- Prophylactic measures include; preexercise warm-up, good intra-session hydration practices, good sleep hygiene, gradual physical conditioning, and improved nutrition.
- Prophylactic medications may be useful; calcium channel blockers, beta-blockers, amitriptyline, or low-dose ergotamine to name a few.

NEUROLOGY

15.4 Jogger's Migraine (Prolonged Exertional Headache)

Clin Sports Med 1992;11:339

Cause: Arises with endurance training, generally low intensity.

Epidem: More common with de-conditioned state, dehydration, hyperthermia, and poor nutrition.

Pathophys: Vascular headache triggered by gradual dehydration and heat accumulation.

Sx:
- Gradual onset of throbbing type headache that is usually generalized or frontal.
- Nausea, vomiting, and visual changes.

Si: Exam usually neg.

Crs: Symptoms may be prolonged in duration.

X-ray: CT or MRI to rule out vascular or structural lesion.

Rx:
- Usually responds to NSAIDs.
- Gradual conditioning program.
- Ensure proper hydration and nutrition.
- Avoid alcohol and caffeine.

15.5 Concussions (Traumatic Brain Injury-TBI)

Am Fam Phys 1999;60:887

Cause: Direct blow to head.

Epidem:
- Approximately 15-20% of high-school football players sustain at least one concussion resulting in 250,000 TBI/yr.
- Fourfold risk of sustaining a second TBI following initial concussion.

- Most common in collision sports but can occur in any sport or activity.

Pathophys:
- Mechanics of injury include both linear and rotational acceleration/deceleration (coup/contra-coup).
- These forces probably result in microscopic axonal shear-strain damage in the pons and midbrain.

Sx:

Acute: Confusion, dizziness, memory loss (event amnesia), loss of consciousness, headache, tinnitus, nausea, vomiting, blurred vision.

Postconcussion: Headache, nausea, memory loss, irritability and personality changes, difficulty sleeping, fatigue, poor school performance, and inattentiveness.

Si:
- Mental status changes including; confusion, long- and short-term memory loss, loss of consciousness.
- Poor motor coordination, poor balance, or vertigo common.
- Cranial nerve evaluation may show deficits with intracranial hemorrhage.

Concussion Grading: There are several grading systems that have been published. These differ substantially in both determination of severity and restriction in return to play. It would seem appropriate to use the more conservative (Colorado Medical Society) for collision sports where the risk of repeat injury is high, and the less restrictive (Cantu) for sports where the risk of re-injury is less.

Table 15.1   Concussion Grading

	Grade 1	Grade 2	Grade 3
Colorado Medical Society (CMS)	No loss of consciousness, with symptoms lasting less than 15 min	No loss of consciousness, with symptoms lasting more than 15 min	Any loss of consciousness
Cantu	No loss of consciousness; posttraumatic amnesia less than 30 min	Loss of consciousness less than 5 min or posttraumatic amnesia greater than 30 min	Loss of consciousness greater than 5 min or posttraumatic amnesia greater than 24 hr

X-ray: CT: Recommended for eval of LOC, seizure, or facial neuro findings to r/o hemorrhage.

Lab:

Neuropsychometric testing: Useful in detecting or following subtle cognitive deficits. These tests are being used frequently, however precise guidance for clinical use remains controversial.

Rx:
- Initial management involves ABCs in the unconscious athlete.
- C-spine protection until evaluated.
- Complete neurologic assessment and special testing as indicated.
- Primary treatment in conscious athlete is protection from re-injury and second impact syndrome through return to play restrictions.
- Pt should be reassessed frequently after injury to ensure no change in neurologic status.
- May be treated symptomatically for headaches and other complaints.

Return to Play:

Table 15.2   Concussion Return to Play Recommendations

	Grade 1	Grade 2	Grade 3
Colorado Medical Society (CMS)	1st Injury: Return to play when asymptomatic for 20 min	1st Injury: Return to play when asymptomatic for 1 wk	1st Injury: Transport to hospital. Return to play 1 mo after injury if asymptomatic for 2 wk
	2nd Injury: Return to play when asymptomatic for 1 wk	2nd Injury: Return to play after asymptomatic for 1 mo	2nd Injury: Terminate season Discourage return
	3rd Injury: Terminate May return in 3 mo	3rd Injury: Terminate season; may return next season	
Cantu	1st Injury: May return to play if asymptomatic	1st Injury: Return after asymptomatic for 1 wk	1st Injury: Wait at least 1 mo; may return then if asymptomatic for 1 wk
	2nd Injury: May return in 2 wk if asymptomatic at that time for 1 wk	2nd Injury: Wait at least 1 mo; may return then if asymptomatic for 1 wk; consider terminating season	2nd Injury: Terminate season; may return next yr if asymptomatic
	3rd Injury: Terminate season; may return next yr if asymptomatic	3rd Injury: Terminate season; may return next yr if asymptomatic	

Postconcussion Syndrome:
- Common constellation of symptoms in the postinjury period lasting from hrs to wks. Include headache, exertional headache, memory and cognition impairment, personality changes (irritability), fatigue, and dizziness.
- Persistent symptoms warrant CT or MRI imaging. Return to play should be restricted until an appropriate period after all postconcussive symptoms have resolved (see Table 15.2).

15.6 Second Impact Syndrome

Clin Sports Med 1998;17:37

Cause:
- A catastrophic brain injury resulting from repetitive concussive injury in the immediate postconcussive period.
- Results in rapid collapse and death.

Epidem: Most commonly reported in boxing and hockey; more common in adolescents.

Pathophys:
- Related to loss of autoregulation of intracranial blood flow leading to dramatic increase in intracranial pressure and herniation.
- Typical pt is involved in a second blow to the head after sustaining a mild concussion.

Sx: Following repetitive blows to the head the pt collapses into a coma that is refractory to medical or surgical intervention.

Si: Coma.

Crs: Typically dies of brainstem herniation resulting from massive edema.

X-ray: MRI or CT demonstrate massive cerebral edema and brainstem herniation.

Rx:
- In reported cases, acute intervention not effective.
- Only effective treatment is prevention.
- "Sideline" physician must be diligent in identifying athletes w even minor head injuries and restrict participation as appropriate.

15.7 Intracranial Hemorrhage

Br J Sports Medicine 1996;30:289

Subarachnoid:

Cause: May be due to direct trauma or may arise atraumatically from vascular anomaly.

Sx:
- Presentation dependent upon volume.
- Large bleed leads to rapid loss of consciousness and death, small bleed may present as gradually worsening and persistent headache.
- Associated symptoms may include visual changes, photophobia, nausea, vomiting, nuchal rigidity, aphasia, dizziness, and cognitive changes.

X-ray: CT scan, MRI, and/or angiography define lesion and source.

Lab: Lumbar puncture can identify ICB.

Rx: These pts should be evaluated by a neurosurgeon.

Epidural:

Cause: Arise from direct blow to head, often associated with skull fracture.

Sx:
- Initial headache, nausea, vomiting, and disequilibrium following head trauma.
- Loss of consciousness follows.

NEUROLOGY

Crs: Death occurs due to intracranial pressure causing herniation.

X-ray: CT or MRI confirms diagnosis.

Rx: Immediate neurosurgical consultation required.

Subdural:

Most common cause of death from head injury in an athlete. Usually associated with immediate and persistent loss of consciousness. Requires immediate neurosurgical consultation.

Upper Extremity Peripheral Neuropathies

Median Nerve

15.8 Carpal Tunnel Syndrome

Neurol Clin 1999;17:407

Cause: Compression of the median nerve as it traverses the carpal tunnel formed by the volar surface of the proximal carpal row, interosseous membrane, and the median retinaculum.

Epidem: Most common compressive neuropathy of the upper extremity.

Pathophys: Inflammation of the flexor tendons results in swelling and increased pressure within the closed space of the carpal tunnel.

Sx:
- Numbness involving mid and distal palmar hand, thumb and index, ring and radial half of the ring finger.
- Pain in the wrist and hand are also common.
- Symptoms may be worse at night and frequently the pt awakens w numbness.
- Frequently complain of weakness or clumsiness in affected hand.

Si:

- Sensory changes in the distribution of the median nerve. Thenar atrophy and motor weakness common.
- Tinel's sign: percussion at the ulnar side of the palmaris longus tendon at the distal flexion crease increases numbness or tingling.
- Phalen's test: holding the wrist in a maximally flexed position produces numbness (Figure 15.1).

Lab: Electromyography and nerve conduction testing are useful in confirming presence of compressive medial neuropathy and determining severity and chronicity of syndrome.

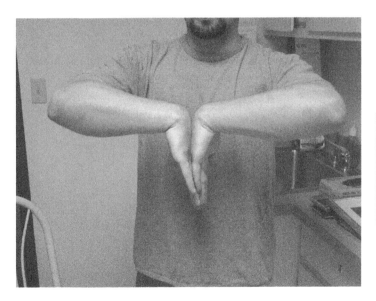

Figure 15.1 Phalen test

Rx:

- Initial treatment includes bracing, oral anti-inflammatories, activity modification.
- Corticosteroid injection: medication is injected beneath the flexor retinaculum at the distal flexion crease on the radial side of the palmaris longus.
- Surgical release of the flexor retinaculum is often required, but does not exclude the possibility of symptom recurrence.

15.9 Pronator Syndrome

Neurol Clin 1999;17:407

Cause: Proximal compressive neuropathy of the medial nerve occurring at the proximal flexor aspect of the forearm.

Epidem: Most common in throwing sports, wt lifters.

Pathophys: Compression occurs at the ligament of Struthers, pronator teres, lacertus fibrosus, or flexor digitorum sublimus.

Sx:

- Complain of numbness in thumb, index, middle, and radial ring finger with activity.
- Associated with forearm flexor compartment pain.
- Usually affects dominant arm.

Si:

- Location of compression can be localized by exam.
- Increased symptoms with resisted elbow flexion (between 120-135°) suggests entrapment at ligament of Struthers.
- Symptoms with flexion of the middle finger suggest entrapment at the sublimus arch.
- Tinel's sign will localize to the level of the lesion.
- Phalen's test will be neg.

Lab: Electromyography and nerve conduction testing are useful in confirming presence of compressive medial neuropathy, and determining severity and chronicity of syndrome.

Rx:

- Relative rest, wrist splinting, oral anti-inflammatory medications (consider pulse corticosteroid such as prednisone 60 mg/d for 6 d).
- Surgical exploration for refractory cases.

15.10 Ulnar Nerve

Neurol Clin 1999;17:463; Neurol Clin 1999;17:447

Cause: Symptoms arise from compression or stretch of nerve usually at elbow (ulnar notch) or hand (Guyon's canal).

Epidem: Most common in cyclists, throwers, racquet sports.

Pathophys: At the elbow, traverses medial epicondyle beneath fascia of the flexor carpi ulnaris. Ulnar neuropathy at the elbow arises from direct trauma, subluxation over the epicondyle, or due to chronic inflammatory changes of the flexor carpi ulnaris. In the wrist and hand, passes between the pisiform and hook of the hamate (Guyon's canal). In the wrist, the symptoms arise from a mass lesion (ganglion), direct trauma, or mechanical factors related to wrist position (cyclists' palsy).

Sx:

- Entrapment at the elbow presents with elbow pain radiating to wrist and 4th and 5th fingers.
- Paresthesias generally involve the ulnar hand and 4th and 5th fingers and are made worse w percussion in the ulnar notch or w maximal elbow flexion.
- Entrapment at Guyon's canal will involve distal paresthesias without motor weakness of the flexors (interosseous muscle may still be affected).

Si: Motor weakness may arise with chronic compression affecting flexor carpi ulnaris, 4th and 5th finger flexors, and the interosseous muscles.

X-ray: Radiographs (AP, lat, carpal tunnel view): evaluate for fractures of the hamate or pisiform.

Lab: Electromyography and nerve conduction testing will usually localize the site of entrapment.

Rx:

At the elbow:
- Relative rest, anti-inflammatories, physical modalities.
- Elbow splint.
- Surgical decompression or transposition.

At the wrist (cyclists' palsy):
- Relative rest, anti-inflammatories for acute symptoms.
- Padded palm gloves, alteration of wrist position w activity.
- Surgical exploration, if symptoms persist.

15.11 Radial Nerve: Radial Tunnel Syndrome

J Hand Surg [Br] 1998;23:617

Cause:
- Entrapment of the posterior interosseous branch of the radial nerve as it passes beneath the fibrous arcade of the supinator.
- Frequently implicated in cases of recalcitrant tennis elbow.

Epidem: Common in racquet sports, golf (lead arm).

Sx:
- Symptoms initially mimic tennis elbow w pain at the lateral elbow.
- This extends into the extensor forearm and may radiate distally.
- Pain is worse with gripping or wrist extension.

Si:
- Tenderness at the radial tunnel (4-6 cm distal to the lateral epicondyle).

- Pain w resisted supination of the wrist.
- Pain w resisted extension of the middle finger (localized to the radial tunnel).

Lab: Electromyography is useful for confirmation.

Rx:

- Initial treatment should include relative rest, wrist splinting, and anti-inflammatory medications.
- Surgical decompression considered with EMG confirmation and refractory symptoms.

Chapter 16

Adolescent and Pediatric Problems

16.1 Spondylolysis

Prim Care 2005;32:201; Ortho Clin North Am 2003;34:461; Phy Sportsmed 2001;29:27; Phy Sportsmed 1996;24:57; Clin Sports Med 1993;12:517

Cause: Fracture of pars interarticularis of the lumbar spine.

Epidem: Prevalence 5% in general population; 43% of LBP in adolescents; 63% among divers; 36% in weight lifters; 33% in wrestlers; 32% in gymnasts; 23% in track and field; 85-90% at L5 and 5-15% at L4.

Pathophys:
- Functional anatomy: the pars interarticularis is the bridge of bone between the superior and inferior facets; the pars is stressed by hyperextension activities.
- These are thought to be stress fractures, but may exist congenitally.

Sx: Back pain aggravated by extension activity (arching back in volleyball, weight lifting, running downhill, the follow-through in a rowing stroke); usually not associated w radicular symptoms.

Si: Usually without palpable back pain; may have tight hamstrings; pain w standing single leg hyperextension (stork test)—pt standing with examiner behind, pt stands on one leg and the examiner assists as the pt hyperextends over the stance leg; pos is unilateral exacerbation of pain on the affected side; no palpable bony tenderness (Figure 16.1).

Crs: Progressive worsening of pain w activity.

Cmplc: Spondylolisthesis (see 16.2).

Diff Dx: Discitis, Sheuermann's (see 16.2), HNP (see 9.2), tumor.

X-ray:
- Plain film oblique view demonstrating lucent line in the neck of the "Scotty dog."
- Bone scan may demonstrate focal signal in the pars.
- SPECT (single photon emission computed tomography) done with the bone scan is very specific in identifying pars lesion.
- MRI may demonstrate signal and or fx of the pars.
- CT will demonstrate completed fx only.

Rx:
- Relative rest for 4-6 wk from offending activity avoiding hyperextension and high impact activity.
- Pain control with ice/heat/NSAIDs.
- Physical therapy focused on hamstring flexibility and abdominal muscle strengthening. Once pain free, may cross train w low impact (bike, swim, deep water run, stairmaster) aerobics and LE wt lifting.
- If sx persist or return early consider longer restriction or immobilization in a TLSO (thoracolumbar spinal orthosis) brace with monthly follow-up. Bracing is discontinued when pt is pain free with daily activities and has a nl exam. At this point, therapy is started for strengthening and stabilization.
- There are arguments that bracing should be the initial treatment for all pts; studies have shown radiographic healing of acute lesions w bracing and activity restriction.
- Refer to orthopedics or a spine specialist for refractory cases of pain despite adequate immobilization, signs of infection or HNP.

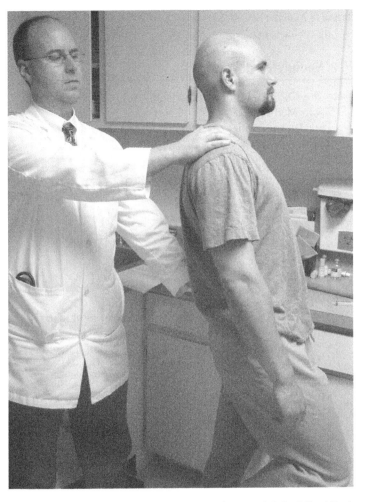

Figure 16.1 Single leg extension test for posterior element pain in back (Stork Test)

Return to Activity: Full ROM with neg stork test; return to impact activity slowly monitoring pain.

16.2 Spondylolisthesis

Prim Care 2005;32:201; Ortho Clin North Am 2003;34:461; Clin Sports Med 2002;21:133; The Low Back Pain Handbook. Philadelphia: Hanley & Belfus, Inc. 1997;331; Pediatric and Adolescent Sports Medicine. Philadelphia: WB Saunders 1994;164

Cause: Anterior slippage of spine.

Epidem:
- 50% of those with bilateral pars defects will develop anterior slippage.
- 90% at L5-S1.
- Runs in families.
- Slippage usually occurs between 9-13 yr.

Pathophys:
- Anterolisthesis involves the anterior movement of the overlying vertebral body on the affect body ie, L5 on S1.
- Causes include bilateral spondylolysis, pars elongation from healed stress fractures, degeneration (seen in the elderly).
- Classification:
  Grade 1: <25% anterior slippage
  Grade 2: 25-50%
  Grade 3: 50-75%
  Grade 4: >100%

Sx: Pain below the beltline aggravated by twisting, extension, or prolonged standing.

Si: May have a "waddling" gait; hamstring tightness, hyperlordosis, pain with extension (stork test, see 16.1); may have neurologic findings (rare, but usually in L5 or S1 distribution); in severe cases of slippage, may palpate a step-off in the spinous processes.

Crs: Variable, but progressive pain with more advanced and progressive slips.

Cmplc: Radiculopathy or HNP (see 9.2).

Diff Dx: Discitis, HNP (see 9.2), compression fx.

X-ray: Lateral L-spine demonstrating anterior slip of one vertebrae on the other.

Rx:

- Asymptomatic:
    <25%: no restrictions on activity with exam and lateral
        L-spine film every 6-12 mo through growth period.
    25-50%: restrict from collision sports or high-risk activities in-
        volving hyperextension or high impact.
    >50% or w progression, surgical stabilization.
- Symptomatic (pain):
    <25%: activity restriction and pain control; part-time bracing,
        if needed w gradual wean and return to activities when
        pain free.
    25-50%: rest and bracing (Boston anti-lordotic); counseling
        against returning to high-risk activities.
    >50%: surgery; other indications for surgery include pain
        >6-12 mo unrelieved by rest or immobilization with any
        grade, progressive slip, neurologic symptoms.

Return to Activity: Good hamstring flexibility; no pain with single leg hyperextension; pt and parents understand risks and will return if increasing symptoms.

16.3 Scheuermann's Kyphosis

Campbell's Operative Orthopedics. 10th ed. St. Louis: Mosby,
    2003;1878; Clin Sport Med 2002;21:133
The Low Back Pain Handbook. St. Louis: Mosby, 1997;336; Major
    Prob Ped 1986;28:52; Pediatric and Adolescent Sports Medicine.
    WB Saunders 1994;170

Cause: Wedging of 3 or more consecutive vertebrae of at least 5° and or kyphosis >35°.

Epidem: 0.4-8.3% of population; most common in boys 13-17 y/o; classic Sheuermann's occurs between T7-T10.

Pathophys:
- Functional anatomy:
  - Lumbar and thoracic vertebral end plates (epiphyses) above and below each vertebral body.
- Developmental collapse of this epiphysis.
- Schmorl's nodes.
  - May be anterior or central.
  - Represent herniation of nucleus pulposis through the end plate.

Sx: Back pain with forward bend; may be nonpainful.

Si: Increased thoracic kyphosis; normal neuro exam.

Crs: Progression is variable.

Cmplc: Chronic pain and deformity (kyphosis).

Diff Dx: Compression fracture, postural problem (round back), discitis, tumor, osteomyelitis.

X-ray: Irregular vertebral end plates, Schmorl's nodes, anterior wedging >5° of 3 or more consecutive thoracic vertebrae or one or more in thoracolumbar Scheuermann's.

Rx:
- Kyphosis <50% without progression:
  - Follow-up x-ray every 4-6 mo.
  - Emphasis on stretching hamstring and pectoralis muscles, lumbar flexion exercises, and spine extensor strengthening.
- Kyphosis >50° brace (TLSO or Milwaukee Brace) worn 16-18 hr/d; low-risk activities are encouraged and can be done w/o brace.

- Surgery if deformity not controlled with bracing or a rigid kyphosis >80°.
- Referral for all cases >35° is prudent.

Return to Activity: Pain-free ROM; no sport activity for 1 yr after surgical fusion for more advanced cases.

16.4 Osteochondritis Dessicans of the Knee (OCD)

Prim Care 2005;32:253; Ortho Clin North Am 2003;34:341; Grainger & Allison Diag Rad 4th ed: London; Churchill Livingstone, Inc. 2001; 2040; Phy Sportsmed 1998;26:31; Clin Sports Med 1997;16:157; Pediatr Clin No Am 1996;43:1067; Sports Medicine: The School-Age Athlete. 2nd ed: Philadelphia; WB Saunders 1996;273

Cause: Cause is currently thought to be multifactorial.

Epidem:
- Approximately 15-30 cases per 100,000.
- Most frequently between 13 to 21 y/o.
- Males are affected at least twice as often as females.
- Bilateral in 20-30% of cases.
- Juvenile and adult onset:
  - Juvenile OCD occurs in pts with open epiphyseal plate.
  - Adult OCD is seen in pts with a closed physes.

Pathophys:
- Exact pathophysiology unknown. The five suggested theories are ischemia, genetic predisposition, abnormal ossification, trauma, and cyclical strain.
- Regardless of the cause the result is a partial or complete separation of a segment of normal hyaline cartilage.
- The plane of separation varies, but is most commonly just below the subchondral plate, creating an osteochondral fragment.
- Typically lesions progress through 4 stages. Intervention at any stage can arrest the process. Staging based on MRI imaging:

Stage 1: compression fx/normal XR.
Stage 2: partially detached; osteochondral fragment.
Stage 3: defect is detached/loose but within underlying cartilage.
Stage 4: defect detached and migrated.

- About 80-85% of cases occur on the medial condyle with the majority classically located on the lateral aspect within the intercondylar notch. The lateral femoral condyle and patella are less commonly affected.

Sx:

- Knee pain, often vague and diffuse.
- Intensity of pain often related to activity level often w swelling.
- If a loose body is present pts may present w catching, locking, or giving way.

Si: May or may not have effusion; thigh atrophy and pos meniscal tests.

Crs:

- The prognosis varies.
- In situ lesions may heal spontaneously or progress to eventually become dislodged, forming a loose body within the joint.
- Skeletally immature pts frequently only require conservative management, while skeletally mature pts or those w a loose body generally require surgical intervention.

Cmplc: OCD in adults is more likely to progress to OA, intra-articular loose bodies, chronic pain, and disability.

Diff Dx: Fracture, neoplasm, ligamentous injury, meniscal injury (see 11.3), retropatellar knee pain (see 11.8).

X-ray:

- Well-delineated lesion in the subchondral bone best seen on tunnel view.

- Bone scans can help with establishing a diagnosis and prognosis since a relationship exists between radionuclide uptake and healing potential.
- MRI is particularly helpful in distinguishing between Stage 2 and 3 lesions.
- Arthroscopy useful to determine size, stability, and site of lesion.

Rx:

- Goal of treatment is to preserve articular cartilage and treatment varies depending on stage of lesion and skeletal maturity.
- Intervention at any stage may arrest process.
- Stage 1 and 2 lesions activity modification, non-wt-bearing and short-term immobilization.
- Stages 3 and 4 lesions should be referred to orthopedics for arthroscopy.
- Refer all pts with loose bodies and/or skeletal maturity.

16.5 Osteochondritis Dessicans (OCD) of the Elbow/Panner's Disease (Osteochondrosis of the Capitellum)

Prim Care 2005;32:253; Clin Sports Med 2004;23:581; DeLee and Drez's Orthopedic Sports Med. 2nd ed. Philadelphia: WB Saunders 2004;1284; Am J Orthop 1998;27:90; Phy Sportsmed 1997;25:85

Cause: Repetitive trauma through throwing or repetitive axial loading in a skeletally immature elbow.

Epidem:

- M>F
- Typically the dominant arm of adolescent baseball players (particularly pitchers) and gymnasts.
- Also seen in weight lifting, racquet sports, and cheerleading.

Pathophys:

- Throwing or repetitive axial loading causes a large tensile force on the medial side of the elbow, as well as a compressive force on the lateral side (radiocapitellar articulation), leading to microfracture and eventual avascular necrosis.
- Usually occurs at the lateral or central portion of the capitellum, although lesions of the trochlea, radial head, and olecranon fossa have also been reported.
- The OCD lesion or fragment of articular surface containing both articular cartilage and subchondral bone may remain in situ or detach and form a loose body.
- Panner's disease (osteochondrosis):
  - Benign, self-limited disorder of the capitellum ossification center. Involves an interference of the blood supply to the epiphysis and is characterized by degeneration, regeneration, and replacement of the ossification center.
  - Not related to repetitive trauma; can occur spontaneously.
  - Most common cause of lateral elbow pain in children <10 y/o.
  - Presentation, radiologic findings, and treatment is similar to OCD.

Sx:

- Decreased athletic performance (decreased velocity and distance of throws).
- Elbow pain with activities.
- Stiffness and inability to fully straighten elbow.
- May progress to repeated locking episodes.

Si:

- Tenderness to palpation in radiocapitellar joint.
- Decreased elbow ROM (normal is full extension or 10° hyperextension to 150° flexion, 90° supination and pronation).
- Occasional swelling and radialhumeral joint crepitus.

Crs:

- Dependent on size and if displacement has occurred. Smaller in situ lesions will typically heal with a break from the offending activity.
- Continued repetitive stress, will lead to progression of disease to include: decreased performance and ROM (flexion, extension, and pronation), loose body formation, early degenerative changes.

Cmplc: Limited function, degenerative arthritis.

Diff Dx: Lateral epicondylitis (see 6.1), biceps tendonitis (insertional) (see 6.10), tumor; infectious or inflammatory arthritis, recent or remote radial head fx. (see 6.6), pin entrapment (see 6.4).

Lab: Normal WBC, ESR; only needed to rule out inflammatory conditions.

X-ray:

- Cystic lesion or radiolucency within the humeral capitellum, may include loose body and hypertrophy of the radial head.
- If plain film is unable to detect osteochondral injury and high index of suspicion, consider MRI or CT arthrogram.

Rx:

- Nondisplaced lesions may heal with rest and protection (avoid throwing, vaulting and floor exercises in gymnastics until pain has resolved and full motion has returned).
- Lesions that are loose or partially detached may be reattached by internal fixation.
- Displaced lesions should be surgically excised.

Apophysitis

16.6 Osgood-Schlatter Disease (OSD)

Ortho Clin North Am 2003;34:405; Phy Sportsmed 1998;26:29;
Pediatric and Adolescent Sports Medicine. Philadelphia: WB
Saunders 1994;320

Cause: Inflammation of the apophysis of the tibial tubercle.

Epidem: Osgood Schlatter's is most common knee complaint in children, with a prevalence of 21% in athletic adolescents; presents in girls 8-13 y/o and boys 10-15; 20-30% occurs bilaterally.

Pathophys: Apophyses are growth centers at the insertion of major tendons and ligaments into bone; poor flexibility and recurrent traction of the muscle-tendon unit causes microfractures of this growth center during the growth spurt.

Sx: Pain at tibia tuberosity with activity.

Si: Painful selling of tibial tuberosity; no joint line tenderness.

Crs: Recurrent pain with increased activity reduced by rest.

Cmplc: Avulsion of tubercle; painful ossicle requiring surgical excision; permanent prominence of the tubercle.

Diff Dx: Patellar tendonitis (see 11.9), tumor proximal tibia, knee OCD (see 16.4), Sinding-Larsen-Johansson (see 16.7), patellofemoral pain syndrome (see 12.8); SCFE (see 16.10), Legg-Calve-Perthes (see 16.11).

X-ray: Lateral radiograph demonstrating fragmentation or irregular ossification of the tibial tubercle.

Rx:
- Relative rest from high-impact activity for short period (1-4 d).
- Ice for pain control (ice massage or apply bag of frozen peas or corn for 20 min after activity).
- Resume activity, as tolerated.

- Hamstring and quad stretching.
- Consider patellar tendon counterforce brace (Cho-Pat or other brands) for activity.
- Consider immobilization or short use of crutches for severe episodes of pain.

Return to Activity: Limited by pain; may need repeated episodes of decreased activity during more active seasons of the yr.

16.7 Sinding-Larsen-Johanssen (SLJ)

Pediatric and Adolescent Sports Medicine. Philadelphia: WB Saunders 1994;325; Clin Sports Med 2002;21:461; Ortho Clin North Am 2003;34:405

Cause: Apophysitis of the inferior pole of the patella.

Epidem: Preteen boys (10-12 y/o).

Pathophys: Persistent traction at the immature inferior patellar pole leading to calcification and ossification.

Sx: Activity related anterior knee pain esp with high impact activities (running and jumping).

Si: Pain, swelling, and tenderness at the inferior pole of the patella; may have hamsting tightness.

Crs: Self-limiting.

Cmplc: Chronic pain, patellar tendon avulsion.

Diff Dx: RPPS (see 11.8), OCD (see 16.4), Osgood-Schlatter (see 16.6); patellar stress fracture, patellar tendinitis.

X-ray: Usually normal or may demonstrate calcification or elongation of the inferior pole of the patella; may demonstrate bipartite patella.

Rx:
- Activity moderation when symptomatic.
- Ice massage (15 min) or application of crushed ice in a bag (or frozen vegetables) for postactivity pain.

- Therapy emphasis on hamstring and quadricep flexibility.
- Prn use of NSAIDs in age-appropriate doses.
- Consider a patellar tendon counterforce brace (Cho-Pat or other brand) or neoprene knee sleeve.
- No injections due to risk of tendon rupture.

Return to Activity: As tolerated, limited by pain.

16.8 Sever's Disease

Ortho Clin North Am 2003;34:405; Pediatric and Adolescent Sports Medicine. Philadelphia: WB Saunders 1994;95; Med Sci Sports Exerc 1999;37:S470

Cause: Calcaneal apophysitis; inflammation and pain in the os calcus apophysis (insertion of Achilles tendon).

Epidem: common in 9-12 y/o range and those involved in high-impact activities (gymnastic, soccer, running).

Pathophys: Apophyses are growth centers at the insertion of major tendons and ligaments into bone; poor flexibility and recurrent traction of the muscle-tendon unit causes microfractures of this growth center during the growth spurt.

Sx: Posterior heel pain with activity.

Si: Posterior heel pain along the sides at the insertion of the Achilles.

Crs: Usually self-limiting with symptoms related to level of impact activity.

Cmplc: Chronic pain; avulsion.

Diff Dx: Calcaneal stress fracture (see 14.20), plantar fasciitis (see 14.19), tarsal tunnel (see 14.22), retrocalcaneal bursitis (see 14.21).

X-ray: Lateral calcaneal view may demonstrate irregular contour of apophysis; consider bone scan or MRI to r/o stress fx.

Rx:
- Relative rest from high-impact activity.
- Ice massage or applied crushed ice in a bag or frozen vegetables in a bag for postactivity pain.
- Prn use of dose-appropriate NSAIDs or Tylenol.
- Aggressive heel cord stretching.
  - Wall stretch of gastroc-soleus: hold 20 sec 5 × per session and repeat 5 ×/d.
- Consider Tulley heel cup for activity.
- Consider PT for modalities.

Return to Activity: As tolerated; good heel cord stretch w slow return to high impact activity.

16.9 Medial Elbow Apophysitis (Little League Elbow)

Ortho Clin North Am 2003;34:405; Pediatric and Adolescent Sports Medicine. Philadelphia: WB Saunders 1994;250

Cause: Throwing in baseball (esp curve balls).

Epidem:
- The term "Little League Elbow" is a group of elbow diagnoses including:
  - Medial epicondylar fragmentation and avulsion or delayed or accelerated apophyseal growth of the medial epicondyle.
  - OCD of the capitellum (see 16.5).
  - Osteochondrosis of the radial head.
  - Flexion contracture of the elbow.
  - Olecranon stress fracture.
- Highly associated with pitch count (> 600/season).
- Increased sx with split finger pitches, increasing age, increased weight, fatigue, poor satisfaction, and playing with multiple teams.
- May also be seen in gymnasts.

Pathophys:
- Apophyses are growth centers at the insertion of major tendons and ligaments into bone.
- Valgus stress from the throwing motion places a stretching stress on the medial elbow.
- The strong ulnar collateral ligament takes origin on the medial epicondyle (epiphysis) and inserts on the ulna.

Sx: Medial elbow pain w activity or at night and with ADLs for more severe cases; try to quantitate throwing (innings pitched, types of pitches, changes in training or game schedule); query for prior or coexistent wrist, shoulder, or back problems.

Si:
- Observe ROM (may have a flexion contracture in the affected elbow for chronic irritation and contracture of the anterior joint capsule):
  - Have pt elevate arms to side with elbows fully extended and compare R to L.
- Observe for atrophy of muscles (flexor group) or hypertrophy of medial epicondyle.
- Tenderness over the medial epicondyle.
- Pain or laxity w valgus stress (see section 6.7):
  - Examiner stabilizes the elbow with one hand with the elbow flexed 90° and then applies a valgus (away from the midline) stress observing for laxity or pain and compares to opposite side.
  - Check for evidence of ulnar nerve subluxation or tenderness (Tinel's) in the ulnar groove of the medial elbow.

Crs: Progressive, if not adequately rested.

Cmplc: Avulsion of medial epicondyle, other components of the "Little League Elbow," loose body.

Diff Dx: Referred pain from neck or shoulder problems, occult fracture.

X-ray:

- Plain films may demonstrate fragmentation, beaking, or enlargement of the medial epicondyle; compare R to L to observe for change; may see a loose body.
- MRI may well demonstrate inflammation of the medial epicondylar apophysis.
- CT usually indicated for evaluation of loose bodies.

Rx:

- Initial rest for 4-6 wk from throwing.
- Ice massage and NSAIDs or Tylenol for pain.
- Splinting for very severe cases (short duration).
- Stretching of anterior joint capsular contractures:
  - Formally through PT or apply heat for 10 min, and then place a small wt in the hand with elbow resting on a table and stretch the anterior joint capsule.
- After 6-8 wk of rest then start strengthening and a very slowly progressive throwing program or other sport activity.

Return to Activity: Pain-free ROM; no pain with valgus stress of the elbow; no laxity; 85% strength; recommended pitch counts by age: 8-10 y/o 52+15; 11-12 y/o 68+18; 13-14 y/o 76+16; no sidearm throwing; focus on fastball and change-up pitches and restrict split finger fastball to >16 y/o.

16.10 Slipped Capital Femoral Epiphysis (SCFE)

CPEM 2002;3:129; Phy Sportsmed 2003;31:39; Phy Sportsmed 1996;24:69; DeLee and Drez's Othopaedic Sports Medicine. 2nd ed: Philadelphia: WB Saunders 2003;1466; Pediatric and Adolescent Sports Medicine. Philadelphia: WB Saunders 1994;281

Cause: Shearing failure of the proximal femoral epiphysis.

Epidem: M>F almost 2:1; bilateral 20-50%; usually 9-16 y/o; obese or tall and thin pts; 4% with have a pos FH.

Pathophys: Weakened physis during the growth spurt; participation in impact activity; onset can be gradual (chronic) or sudden (acute).

Sx: Painful wt-bearing or limp with pain isolated to anterior groin, thigh or knee; in chronic cases, pain is dull and intermittent, lasting 3 wks or more; in acute cases, pain is sharp and persistent with more instability.

Si: Painful ROM with limited internal rotation (IR); may have shortening of the affected limb; pos Whitman's sign (passive flexion of the hip by the examiner causes the limb to abduct and externally rotate as the thigh moves toward the abdomen).

Crs: Progressive with either early complete slip or chronic silent slip.

Cmplc: AVN of the femoral head (see 10.2); chondrolysis of the articular cartilage; premature hip OA for chronic silent cases.

Diff Dx: Legg-Calvé-Perthes (see 16.11), toxic synovitis (see 16.12), tumor in the femur, adductor strain (see 10.5).

X-ray: AP and frog-leg lateral demonstrating slippage to the epiphysis, widening of the physis (as compared to the opposite side).

Rx: When suspicious, place the patient non-wt-bearing immediately until is or is not confirmed; immediate referral to orthopedics for pinning.

Return to Activity: When cleared by orthopedics; limit activity until several mo after internal fixation devices have been removed (usually done when there is evidence of physeal fusion).

16.11 Legg-Calvé-Perthes (LCP)

CPEM 2002;3:118, CPEM 2002;3:129; Phy Sportsmed 1996;24:69; Pediatric and Adolescent Sports Medicine. Philadelphia: WB Saunders 1994;288; Major Problems Ped 1986;28:77

Cause: Interrupted blood supply to the femoral epiphysis.

Epidem: Usually 4-8 y/o; boys 1:750 and girls 1:3700; familial tendency.

Pathophys:

Stages of disease:
1. Edema of synovium and joint capsule (1-6 wks).
2. Necrosis of femoral epiphysis (several mo to 1 yr).
3. Regeneration and resorption (1-3 yrs): granulation tissue replacing necrotic bone and development of immature bony matrix.
4. Repair: new, normal bone generation.

Sx: Painful limping child; pain from anterior groin to the knee.

Si: Limited IR, Ext, abduction; may have thigh atrophy.

Crs: Depends on the age of onset/diagnosis and percent involvement of the femoral head; younger children with <50% involvement do the best.

Cmplc: Accelerated OA of the hip.

Diff Dx: SCFE (see 16.10), toxic synovitis (see 16.12), femoral tumor.

X-ray:

Radiograph:
• Sclerotic or collapsed epiphysis.

Bone scan:
• Identify avascularity of the femoral epiphysis (head).

MRI:
• Can identify early cases where radiograph may be normal.

Rx: Refer to orthopedics; management may include close observation, bed rest, nonsurgical (abduction bracing or casting), and surgical.

Return to Activity: Restriction of high-impact activity until well into Stage 4 of the healing process; return base on recommendation of orthopedics.

16.12 Toxic Synovitis of the Hip

CPEM 2002;3:129; Major Problems Ped 1986;28:52; Phy Sportsmed 1996;24:69; Am Fam Phys 1996;54:1587

Cause: Postviral synovitis.

Epidem: The most common cause in hip pain in children <10 y/o; average age 5.9 yrs; M:F 2:1.

Pathophys: Etiology unknown.

Sx: Recent URI with c/o limp or inability to walk and low-grade temp.

Si: Temp up to 101°; painful ROM with leg held in flexion and abduction.

Crs: Self-limiting.

Cmplc: LCP (see 16.11).

Diff Dx: Septic arthritis, JRA, early LCP (see 16.11); SCFE (see 16.10), femoral tumor.

Lab: CBC and ESR to r/o septic arthritis (should be normal); consider referral for arthrocentesis and joint fluid eval.

X-ray: Radiographs, MRI, bone scan all WNL.

Rx: Close observation; consider referral for advanced imaging (MRI) or the orthopedics for evaluation and/or arthrocentesis.

Return to Activity: Pain-free ROM and normal gait with walk and run; consider f/u eval with radiographs in 2-3 mo to r/o LCP.

16.13 Salter Harris Fractures

Pediatric and Adolescent Sports Medicine. Philadelphia: WB Saunders 1994;149

Cause: Usually acute trauma, but may be an overuse injury.

Epidem: 15-20% of long bone injuries involve the physis; UE:LE is
2:1; M>F is 2:1; peak incidence 11 y/o in girls and 12-13 y/o in
boys; distal radius is the most common (¹/₃ of all injuries), phalangeal #2 and distal tibia #3; physeal disruptions about the knee
are only 2%, but represent >50% of all growth arrest problems.

Pathophys: Physis most susceptible to shear forces and is weaker than
both bone and tendon/ligaments; other causes of injury include
frostbite and osteomyelitis.

Sx: Acute injury with pain.

Si: Isolated pain over the appropriate epiphysis.

Crs: Depends on classification, involved joint, and diagnosis (Figure
16.2):

Salter Harris I—transphyseal separation w no osseous injury.

Salter Harris II—transphyseal separation w metaphyseal fracture
(away from the joint space).

Salter Harris III—transphyseal injury w epiphyseal fracture (fracture toward the joint space).

Salter Harris IV—transphyseal injury w metaphaseal and epiphyseal fracture.

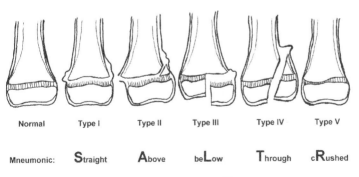

| Normal | Type I | Type II | Type III | Type IV | Type V |

Mneumonic: **S**traight **A**bove be**L**ow **T**hrough c**R**ushed

Figure 16.2 Salter-Harris classification of epiphyseal fractures

Salter Harris V—crush of the physis (epiphyseal plate).
Grades I-III have the best prognosis, IV and V the worst
prognosis.

Cmplc: Growth arrest or bony bridges causing bowing of the bone.

Diff Dx: Strain or sprain, tumor.

X-ray: Plain radiograph may demonstrate widening or shift of the epiphysis w or w/o fracture of the epiphysis or metaphysis.

Rx: Cast or brace immobilization; depending on the affected joint, consider orthopedic referral; management depends on the comfort level and experience of the provider.

Return to Activity: Pain-free ROM w/o pain over the physis or w stressing.

Chapter 17

Cardiovascular Problems

17.1 Exercise-Associated Collapse (EAC)/Syncope

Am Fam Phys 1999;60:2001; Phy Sportsmed 2003;31:23; Clin Auton Res 2004;14S:1-26; Phy Sportsmed 2005;33:28

Causes: Exercise (see Diff Dx).

Epidem:
- Exertional-related syncope represents only a minority (3-20%) of all syncope.
- 1 in 20,000 athletes presenting w syncope has a serious cardiac condition.
- In one study, 85% of EAC occurred after completion of an event. The 15% of EAC which occurred *before* completion were more likely to have an organic etiology.

Pathophys:

Syncope: sudden and temporary loss of consciousness associated w a loss of postural tone.

Exercise-related syncope:
- Syncopal episode occurring during or in the immediate post-exertional period.
- Can signal sudden death and warrants thorough investigation.

Exercise-associated collapse (EAC): broadens the definition and includes athletes who are unable to stand/walk unaided due to lightheadedness, faintness, dizziness, or syncope. It specifically excludes orthopedic injuries. It is most commonly caused by postural hypotension.

Postural hypotension:
- During exercise, an increase in stroke volume (SV) increases cardiac output.
- Muscle contractions are crucial in maintaining venous return and end-diastolic volume (EDV).
- After exercise, lack of muscular contractions decreases EDV and SV.
- This causes a reflex vagal response, leading to vasodilatation, bradycardia, and, hence, hypotension.
- Severe postural hypotension may lead to neurocardiogenic syncope.

Sx:
- Must differentiate between true syncope vs collapse from exhaustive effort, heat injuries, or metabolic conditions (hypoglycemia, hyponatremia):
  - True syncope elicits a history of quick recovery.
  - Collapse due to exhaustive effort usually presents with prolonged periods of semiconsciousness.
- Determine timing of syncopal event in relation to event:
  - Orthostatic hypotension *after* exercise is more benign.
  - Sudden loss of consciousness *during* exercise is ominous (suggests cardiac or arrhythmic etiology).
- Other prodromal symptoms should be elucidated: palpitations (suggesting arrhythmia), chest pain (ischemia, aortic dissection), wheezing/pruritus (anaphylaxis).
- Elicit history of high-risk behaviors, eating disorders, murmurs, medications, and family history of sudden death.

Si:

Vitals signs:
- For on-site events: vital signs, check rectal temperature to r/o heat injuries, and consider testing for sodium and/or glucose levels to r/o hyponatremia and hypoglycemia.

- Office setting: orthostatic blood pressures and BP in arm and leg.

Neuro exam:
- Mental status and ability to walk, especially for on-site events.
- Mental status changes indicate a more serious condition, such as heat stroke or hyponatremia.

Assess for features of Marfan's syndrome (Med Sci Sport Exerc 1998;30:S387):
- Tall, thin stature with disproportionately long arms:
  - Arm span to height ratio >1.05.
- Unusually long lower half of body:
  - Upper-to-lower segment ratio <0.85.
- Long, double-jointed fingers; elongated thumb:
  - Wrist sign: thumb and little finger overlaps considerably when wrapped around wrist.
  - Thumb sign: apposed thumb across palm extends beyond ulnar margin.
- Curvature of the spine (scoliosis).
- Chest wall abnormalities (pectus excavatum or pectus carinatum).
- Murmur of MVP, MR, AR/AI.

Cardiac exam: W auscultation in supine, standing and squatting positions. Document murmurs, clicks, gallops, and pathological splits.
- Systolic murmurs that accentuate w standing suggests HCM.

Crs: Benign course if found to be related to postural hypotension. However, syncope can be a precursor to sudden cardiac death and should be thoroughly investigated.

Cmplc: Seizures, sudden cardiac death.

Diff Dx:
- Neurocardiogenic syncope from postural hypotension (most common).
- Supraventricular tachyarrhythmias.

- Hypertrophic cardiomyopathy (see 17.3).
- Myocarditis/pericarditis (see 17.4).
- Valvular heart disease (Aortic stenosis, MVP, see 17.5).
- Long QT syndrome (see 17.6).
- Coronary artery anomalies.
- Atherosclerotic coronary artery disease.
- Right ventricular dysplasia.
- Exertional hyponatremia (see 22.3).
- Hyperthermia, heat stroke (see 2.8).
- Hypoglycemia.
- Hyponatremia.
- Seizure.

Lab:

- Chemistries: electrolytes, glucose, BUN/CR, CPK (heat injuries, CAD).
- Drug screen, if suspected illicit drug use.
- EKG: r/o long QT, pre-excitation (WPW), LVH, RVH, ischemia.
- GXT: perform after echo. Should be sport-specific, reproduce conditions that led to syncopal event.
- Other special tests: Holter/event monitor (arrhythmias), EP studies (WPW, pre-excitation), EEG (seizures).
- Tilt table testing: not useful in trained athletes; 2° high false pos.

X-ray:

Echo: If clinically warranted, can assess left ventricular function/size (HCM), PA pressures (RV dysplasia), valvular diseases (MVP), coronary artery anomalies (left coronary ostium).

Rx:

- Postural hypotension/neurocardiogenic:
  - Acute, on-site events: place athlete in supine position, elevate legs, and administer oral rehydration until vital signs are stable.

- Chronic events: avoid dehydration and consider β-blockers, disopyramide, SSRI, fludrocortisone.
- Hypertrophic cardiomyopathy (see 17.3).
- Myocarditis (see 17.4).
- SVT: consider ablation.

Return to Activity:
- If history, physical, EKG, and selected lab tests are diagnostic/suggestive and is:
  1) Potentially life threatening → restriction and referral.
  2) Non-life threatening → treat or evaluate/refer, as indicated.
- If history, physical, EKG, and selected lab tests are unexplained; restriction from activity and perform Echo/GXT:
  - Referral if Echo/GXT is diagnostic.
  - Reassurance if normal Echo/GXT with reassuring clinical features (postexertional, nonrecurrent, normal FH, normal cardiac exam.
  - Referral if normal/nondiagnostic Echo/GXT w suggestive clinical features.

17.2 Hypertension

J Am Coll Cardiol 1994;24:885; Jama 2003;289:2560, JNV VII, NIH No. 03-5233; 2003; Med Sci Sports Exerc 2004;36:533

Cause:

Primary (95%): essential hypertension.

Secondary (5%): Coarctation of the aorta, Cushing's syndrome, hyperaldosteronism, hypercalcemia, hyperthyroidism, pheochromocytoma, renal artery stenosis, renal parenchymal disease, various drugs.

Epidem: Occurs in 24-29% of the general adult population, and is the most common cardiovascular condition in competitive athletes (Table 17.1).

Table 17.1 Hypertension Classification by Age

	Normal	Pre-HTN	HTN (Stage 1)	HTN (Stage 2)
Children 6-9 y/o*				
Systolic	<110-114	110-117	119-130	≥126-130 (129)**
Diastolic	<70-75	70-79	80-92	≥87-92 (84)
Children 10-12 y/o*				
Systolic	<115-120	115-122	124-136	≥132-136 (134)
Diastolic	<75-76	75-80	85-94	≥91-94 (89)
Adolescents 13-15 y/o*				
Systolic	<120	120-130	131-143	≥138-143 (149)
Diastolic	<77-79	77-82	86-96	≥94-96 (94)
Adolescents 16-17 y/o*				
Systolic	<120	120-135	139-148	≥146-148 (159)
Diastolic	<80	80-86	89-99	≥97-99 (99)
Adults ≥18 y/o				
Systolic	<120	120-139	140-159	≥160 (180)
Diastolic	<80	80-89	90-99	≥100 (110)

*Calculated at 50th percentile for height; combined age ranges.
Normal: < 90th percentile for age.
Pre-HTN: 90-95th percentile for age.
Stage 1 HTN: 95-99th percentile, plus 5 mm Hg.
Stage 2 HTN: > 99th percentile, plus 5 mm Hg.
More detail, see Peds 114;2004:555.
**Values in parentheses represent classification for severe HTN by the 26th Bethesda Conference.
Classification: JACC 1994;24:886; Jama 2003;289:250; JNC VII; Peds 2004;114:555

Pathophys: Increased total peripheral resistance, which is mediated by plasma epinephrine and norepinephrine in conjunction with the effects of the renin-angiotensin system. The microvascular trauma is thought to be the cause of end-organ damage.

Sx: Usually asymptomatic, but chest pains, dyspnea, orthopnea, poor exercise tolerance may be present. Elicit family history, medication uses, tobacco, ETOH, and illicit drug use.

Si:

Measurement of BP (JNC VII):
- Pt quietly seated in chair with both feet on floor for 5 min and arm supported at heart level.
- No tobacco, caffeine, or exercise within 30 min of measurement.
- Bladder of cuff encircles at least 80% of pt's arm.
- Two or more measurements, average.
- 24-hr ambulatory monitoring may be required to diagnose white-coat and episodic HTN.

Signs of end-organ damage or secondary causes:
- Hypertensive retinopathy, thyromegaly, arterial bruits (esp renal), peripheral pulses, S4 gallop.

Crs: Chronic elevated BPs cause microvascular trauma. This significantly increases the risk of coronary artery disease and left ventricular hypertrophy, increasing the risk of heart failure.

Cmplc: Renal failure, blindness, strokes and TIAs, coronary artery disease, congestive heart failure, dilated cardiomyopathy, hypertrophic cardiomyopathy, and aneurysms.

Lab:

All HTN pts:
- Hematocrit, electrolytes (BUN/Cr, K^+, Ca^{++}, glucose), lipid profile.
- Urinalysis to r/o proteinuria.
- EKG to r/o LVH.

Exercise stress test (GXT) (Med Sci Sports Exerc 2004;36:533):
- May be appropriate to evaluate for those at high risk (history of CAD, diabetes, and/or renal disease or other target organ disease) engaging in moderate intensity exercise (40 − 60% VO_2R).
- Consider for pts engaging in hard or very hard exercise (intensity >60% VO_2R).

X-ray: Echocardiogram to assess for LVH, other tests to r/o secondary HTN.

Rx:

Lifestyle modifications (JNC VII):
- Weight loss, if overweight.
- DASH diet (high fruits and vegetables, lower saturated fats).
- Limit dietary sodium <2.4 gm/d.
- Increase aerobic physical activity (at least 30 min most d of the wk).
- Limit ETOH intake—no more than 1 oz per day (2-12 oz beers, 2 glasses of wine, or 2 mixed drinks) for men, and 0.5 oz for women.

Exercise (Med Sci Sports Exerc 2004;36:533):
- Dynamic activity in hypertensive pts shown to reduce systolic/diastolic BP by 7.4/5.8 mm Hg, respectively in meta-analysis.
- Recommendations: FITT:
  - Frequency: preferably all d of wk.
  - Intensity: moderate-intensity (40 − 60% of VO_2R).
  - Time: ≥30 min of continuous or accumulated physical activity per d.
  - Type: primarily endurance physical activity supplemented by resistance exercise.

Pharmacologic: When lifestyle modification fails to control blood pressure or patient presents with Stage 2 HTN, pharmacologic therapy is indicated. The sports medicine physician must remain conscious of the limitations set forth by the different governing bodies of athletics:
- Angiotensin converting enzyme (ACE) inhibitors:
  - Preferred initial agent for competitive athletes and highly active patients, especially those with diabetes.
  - Use with caution in women because of the teratogenic potential in a developing fetus.

- Ca-channel blockers:
  - Another preferred agent for highly active pts, especially the dihydropyridines.
  - Verapamil and diltiazem should be avoided secondary to their neg inotropic and chronotropic effects on the heart.
- Angiotensin-II receptor blockers (losartan, valsartan):
  - No definitive data in athletes, but felt to be similar to ACE inhibitors.
- Diuretics:
  - Thiazide diuretics are the preferred initial agent (JNC VII).
  - Diuretics, however are not a good choice for endurance athletes due to side effect profile.
  - BANNED by IOC and NCAA.
- β-blockers:
  - The cardio-selective β-blockers (atenolol, metoprolol) are the drugs of choice in the nonendurance athlete and those with CAD.
  - Not recommended for endurance athletes due to decreased aerobic activity.
  - BANNED by IOC and NCAA.
- Central α-receptor agonist (clonidine, methyldopa):
  - No known neg side effects in exercise.
  - The side effects of fatigue, drowsiness, dry mouth, and post-exercise hypotension are not well-tolerated by athletes.
- α-1 receptor blockers (prazosin, terazosin):
  - Decrease peripheral vascular resistance. Best choice for the active patient with benign prostatic hypertrophy.
- Direct vasodilators (hydralazine, minoxidil):
  - Cause a direct vasodilatation thereby lowering blood pressures, which in turn, causes a reflex tachycardia that may not be tolerated by some athletes.

Return to Activity (J Am Coll Cardiol 1994;24:885; Peds 1997;99:637):
- Risk of MI are increased with strenuous static activity due to immediate pressor effect—especially pts with known or occult CAD.

Table 17.2   Classification of Sports

	A. Low Dynamic	B. Moderate Dynamic	C. High Dynamic
I. Low Static	Billiards, bowling, cricket, curling, golf, riflery	Baseball, softball, table tennis, tennis (doubles), volleyball	Badminton, cross-country skiing (classic technique, field hockey, orienteering, race-walking, racquetball, running (long distance), soccer, squash, tennis (singles)
II. Moderate Static	Archery, auto racing, diving, equestrian, motorcycling	Fencing, field events (jumping), figure skating, football (American), rodeoing, rugby, running (sprint), surfing, synchronized swimming	Basketball, ice hockey, cross-country skiing (skating technique), football (Australian rules), lacrosse, running (middle distance), swimming, team handball
III. High Static	Bobsledding, field events (throwing), gymnastics, karate/judo, luge, sailing, rock climbing, waterskiing, weight lifting, windsurfing	Body building, downhill skiing, wrestling	Boxing, canoeing/kayaking, cycling, decathlon, rowing, speed skating

- Although inherently logical, little data exists showing exercise increases the risk for sudden death or progression of hypertensive disease.
- Classification of hypertension has changed, however the recommendations by the 26th Bethesda Conference in 1994 is based on older classifications for children and adults.
- General considerations:
  - Hypertension that is well controlled without evidence of target organ disease, is not a contraindication to competitive activity.
  - Restrict athletes with severe hypertension (>180/110 in adults, >99th percentile in children) particularly from high static sports (see Table 17.2: classes IIIA to IIIC) until HTN controlled and in the absence of target organ damage.
  - Hypertension <180/110 (<99th percentile for children) without CV disease and target organ damage is not a contraindication to competitive sports.
- Classification of sports (J Am Coll Cardiol 1994;24:864).

17.3 Hypertrophic Cardiomyopathy (HCM)

Jama 2002;287:1308; J Am Coll Cardiol 2003;42:1687; Lancet 2004; 363:1881

Cause: Primarily an autosomal dominant genetic disorder of the myocardial contractile unit.

Epidem:
- Most common cause of sudden cardiac death in athletes less than 35 y/o.
- Found in 0.1-0.2% of the general population.

Pathophys:
- Thickened left ventricular wall thickness, which causes an outflow tract obstruction.

- Reduced compliance causes poor ventricular filling.
- Large ventricular mass may outstrip coronary blood supply.

Sx: Usually asymptomatic. Dyspnea, chest pain, palpitations, syncope, lightheadedness.

Si:

- Harsh systolic murmur that gets louder with standing or during Valsalva. Heard best at the left sternal border or apex, and decrease with squatting.
- Paradoxical splitting of S2.
- Double or triple apical impulse.
- Bifid carotid pulse ($^2/_3$ of pts).

Crs (Nejm 2000;342:1778):

- 40% are asymptomatic and are at low risk for sudden death.
- Mild hypertrophy (<19 mm): rate of sudden death <3% in 20 yrs.
- Severe hypertrophy (>30 mm): rate of sudden death >40% in 20 yrs.

Cmplc: Sudden cardiac death, syncope, ventricular arrhythmias, Afib and/or flutter.

Diff Dx: Coronary artery disease, "athlete's heart," hypertensive heart disease, valvular heart disease, pericardial abnormalities.

Lab:

- ECG abnormal in 75-95% of HCM (ST abnormalities, Q-waves, LVH).
- GXT to screen for BP response, PVCs and arrhythmias, if diagnosis confirmed with Echo.
- 24-48 hr holter to screen for arrhythmias, if diagnosis confirmed with Echo.

X-ray:

- CXR recommended to rule out pulmonary disease.
- Echocardiography measurement of left ventricular wall thickness:

- >15mm: consistent with HCM.
- 13-14 mm: "grey zone" may be consistent with "athlete's heart."
- <12 mm: normal.

Rx: Depends on risk factors and if symptomatic. Risk factors include:
1. Symptomatic.
2. Pos family history of sudden death.
3. Sustained/prolonged ventricular tachycardia.
4. Marked outflow tract gradient.
5. Substantial hypertrophy.
6. Left atrial enlargement.
7. Hypotensive BP response during exercise.

Asymptomatic at low risk: Defined as pts w/o or w mild symptoms and none of the above risk factors.
- β-blockers, verapamil, disopyramide often widely prescribed, but no evidence for effectiveness exists.

Asymptomatic at high risk: Defined as pts w/o or with mild symptoms and with + risk factors;
- Medications (β-blockers, verapamil, disopyramide) are highly controversial for prevention of sudden death.
- Implantable cardiac defibrillator (ICD) for prevention of sudden death.
  - Strongly consider in high-risk pts, especially with >30 mm of wall thickness, prior cardiac arrest, sustained VT.

Symptomatic (CHF, Afib, syncope):
- β-blocker—decrease heart rate and increase passive ventricle filling and decreasing myocardial oxygen consumption.
- Verapamil—decreases left ventricular outflow obstruction by improved filling.
- Disopyramide: decreases gradient via neg ionotropic properties.

- Amiodorone: for Afib.
- Administer diuretics and vasodilators w caution.

Surgical/interventional: For pts failing medical management or for severe obstructive outflow gradient (>50 mm):
- Left ventricular myotomy and myectomy to reduce outflow gradient.
- Alcohol septal ablation is a promising alternative and has shown to reduce outflow gradients similar to surgical myotomy-myectomy.
- DDD pacing generally not recommended as primary treatment, but may be nonsurgical option for those >65 y/o.

Return to Activity: Athletes with unequivocal diagnosis of HCM should only participate in class 1A sports (see Table 17.2).

17.4 Myocarditis

Curr Sports Med Rep 2003;2:65; Cardiol Rev 2001;9:88; J Am Coll Cardiol 1994;24:864

Cause: Most common cause is viral (50% coxsackie B). Etiologies can generally be divided into infectious (HIV, Lyme, HSV, Chagas, etc) and noninfectious (lupus, sarcoidosis, drug toxicity, etc).

Epidem: Myocardial inflammation found in 1-4% of autopsies and up to 20% in young adults presenting with sudden death.

Pathophys: Inflammatory infiltration of the myocardium with necrosis and/or degeneration of adjacent myocytes not consistent with ischemia.

Sx: Most are asymptomatic. Three classic presentations:
1. Athlete with chest pain, dyspnea, and exercise intolerance is most common.
2. Healthy athlete with CHF symptoms (DOE, orthopnea, PND).
3. Syncope, EAC, sudden death. Often can elicit history of a viral prodrome.

Si: Tachycardia in setting of fever, tachypnea, pulsus alternans, signs of CHF (S3 gallop, distended neck veins, peripheral edema). May hear friction rub if pericardium involved.

Crs: Three general courses:
1. Full recovery (majority of cases).
2. 10-30% progress to dilated cardiomyopathy (10-30%).
3. 10% have progressive clinical deterioration (leading to death or cardiac transplant).

Cmplc: Sudden cardiac death 2° arrhythmia, biventricular failure, pericarditis, and ventricular arrhythmias.

Diff Dx: Cardiomyopathy, acute MI, valvular heart disease, pulmonary embolism.

Lab:
- Elevated troponin T/I, increased CK with elevated MB fraction, ESR, CRP, and WBC. Consider viral titers and other specific labs to determine causative organism.
- EKG: sinus tachycardia, diffuse, nonspecific ST-T wave changes.
- Biopsy of myocardium for those not responding to treatment.

X-ray:
- CXR: enlargement of cardiac silhouette.
- Echo: dilated hypokinetic chambers, segmental wall motion abnormalities, pericardial effusion.

Rx:
- General supportive care, treat underlying cause.
- Manage CHF with diuretics, ACE inhibitors, digoxin, β-blockers (if hemodynamically stable).
- Steroids, NSAIDs, IVIG, and other immunosuppresants controversial.

Return to Activity (J Am Coll Cardiol 1994;24:864):
- Restrict all physical activity for ~6 mo after onset of clinical signs.

- Undergo full cardiovascular evaluation before returning to activity, including assessment of ventricular function with radionucleotide angiography or Echo.
- Return to play when ventricular function and cardiac dimensions return to normal and ambulatory monitoring reveals no clinically significant arrhythmias.

17.5 Mitral Valve Prolapse (MVP)

Phy Sportsmed 1996;24:78; J Am Coll Cardiol 1994;24:882; J Am Coll Cardiol 1998;32:486

Cause: Autosomal dominant disorder of collagen organization affecting the mitral valve leaflets.

Epidem:
- Most common valvular heart disease, affecting 3-6% of population.
- Increased incidence seen with Ehlers-Danlos syndrome, Marfan's syndrome, and other connective tissue disorders.

Pathophys: Structural abnormality (leaflet thickening with elongation and myxomatous degeneration) that causes substantial protrusion of the valve into the left atrium during systole (MSSE 1994; 26(10)Suppl:S261).

Sx: Palpitations, dizziness, and syncope; chest pain, fatigue, panic attacks.

Si:
- Midsystolic click before a mid to late systolic murmur:
  - Accentuated when the pt is standing.
  - Diminished with squatting.
- Narrow AP chest diameter.

Crs: Most have benign prognosis. Gradual progression of mitral regurgitation may subsequently lead to LV dysfunction and heart failure.

Cmplc: Cardiac arrhythmias, mitral regurgitation, TIA and CVA secondary to emboli, sudden death secondary to cardiac arrhythmia, infective endocarditis, pulmonary hypertension. Higher risk in pts w valvular deformity and/or regurgitation.

Lab: TSH to look for thyroid abnormalities, 24-hr holter to r/o arrhythmias, GXT to monitor exercise tolerance.

X-ray:
- Echo:
  - Anterior and posterior leaflets bulging in systole is diagnostic.
  - Valvular deformity or regurgitation can risk stratify pts.
- Stress Echo for moderate-high risk pts.

Rx:
- Low risk (MVP without valvular deformity or regurgitation):
  - Echo q 5 yrs.
  - Education and reassurance.
  - Palpitations: dietary changes (avoid stimulants), β-blockers, regular exercise.
- Mild risk (MVP with valvular deformity, but no regurgitation):
  - Echo q 2-3 yrs.
  - Oral ABX prophylaxis for SBE.
  - Palpitations: treat as above.
- Moderate risk (MVP with valvular deformity, and mild regurgitation):
  - Echo q 2-3 yrs.
  - Oral ABX prophylaxis for SBE.
  - Palpitations: treat as above.
- High risk (MVP w valvular deformity and moderate-severe regurgitation):
  - Echo q 1 yr.
  - As w moderate risk, closely monitor function and replace valve when necessary.

Return to Activity: Restrict to Class 1A sports (see Table in 17.2) in pts with MVP and one or more of the following (MSSE 1994;26(10)Suppl:S261):

- History of syncope, documented to be arrhythmogenic in origin.
- Family history of sudden death associated w MVP.
- Repetitive forms of sustained and nonsustained supraventricular tachyarrhythmias or complex ventricular arrhythmias, particularly if exaggerated by exercise.
- Moderate to marked mitral regurgitation.
- Prior embolic event.

    All others *without* above criteria may engage in full competitive sports.

17.6 Long QT Syndrome (LQTS)

Cardiol Rev 2004;12:222; Jama 2003;289:2041

Cause: Genetic disorder of variable penetrance. Mapped to 7 LQT genes on 6 chromosomes; LQT_1 and LQT_2 most common subtypes.

Epidem: 1 per 5,000-10,000.

Pathophys: Ion channel dysfunction affecting the cardiac potassium and sodium channels.

Sx:

- Syncope, seizure-like activity and sudden death provoked by exercise or arousal-type emotions (sudden loud noise, alarm clocks).
- Family history of seizure, SIDS, syncope, sudden death.

Si: None.

Crs:

- 50-70% 10-yr mortality rate in untreated pts.
- Sudden death in 20% of actively symptomatic (syncopal) pts.

Cmpl: Syncope and sudden death (presenting symptom in 30% of cases).

Lab:
- Chemistries, to r/o electrolyte abnormalities.
- EKG:
  - QTc usually >0.46 sec.
  - QTc between 0.44-0.46 sec is nondiagnostic.
  - T-wave alternans, notched T-waves.
- GXT: can differentiate nondiagnostic EKGs if:
  - QTc prolongs during recovery phase after exercise.
  - Provokes diagnostic arrhythmia.

Diff Dx: Acquired QT prolongation (medications and electrolyte disturbances), neurocardiogenic syncope, seizures.

Rx:
- β-blockers are the mainstay of treatment for symptomatic pts. Associated with decreased syncope and sudden death.
  - Treatment for asymptomatic pts is controversial.
- Implantable cardiac defibrillators (ICD) is another treatment option, especially those with recurrent syncope despite β-blocker treatment.
- Cardiac pacing and left cardiac sympathetic denervation are options for those intolerant to β-blockers.

Return to Play: Restrict all pts w confirmed long QT syndrome from all competitive sports.

Chapter 18

Issues Unique to the Female Athlete

18.1 Exercise-Associated Amenorrhea

Med Clin N Amer 1994;78:345

Cause: Multifactorial including excessive training, low body wt/low body fat, emotional stress, physical stress of training—all of which lead to suppression of the HPA axis.

Epidem:
- 2-5% of general population.
- 3.4-66% of athletic women, depending on chosen sport.
- Most common in endurance sports (running, XC skiing, triathlon), dancers, gymnasts.

Pathophys:

Exercise-associated amenorrhea related to suppression of GnRH from hypothalamus resulting in reduced LH, estradiol, prolactin, and cortisol release. Should consider other causes (luteal phase dysfunction, polycystic ovarian syndrome, anovulatory amenorrhea).

Primary amenorrhea: failure to reach menarche by 16 y/o.

Secondary amenorrhea: Loss of regular cycle for 3-6 mo after establishing a normal menstrual cycle.

Sx:
- Irregular or absent menstrual cycle for 3-6 mo.
- Failure to reach menarche by 16 y/o.

- Diet and wt history usually reveals below IBW, history of significant wt loss.

Si:

- Body fat assessment: <10-15% concerning although not definitive.
- Pelvic exam: enlarged uterus, ovaries, or adnexal masses.
- Should conduct PAP smear and STD w/u as indicated by history.

X-ray:

- Heel ultrasound: Screening study for bone loss in long-standing amenorrhea.
- DEXA scan: More sensitive and specific test for assessing degree of bone loss in osteoporosis. These tests should be considered in the initial workup of these athletes.

Lab:

- HCG: R/o pregnancy.
- TSH: R/o hypo/hyperthyroidism.
- Prolactin: Evaluate for microadenoma or idiopathic prolactinemia.
- FSH/LH: Typically low in hypothalamic dysfunction.
- Estradiol: Confirmatory in unopposed estrogen states.

Crs: Bone loss may be seen in 3-6 mo with irreversible losses in 24-36 mo.

Rx:

- Reduced training intensity and volume: 10% reduction has been associated with resumption of normal menses.
- Increased % body fat: All EAA cases should receive nutritional counseling by nutritionist familiar with athlete care.
- Estrogen replacement:
  - In EAA, bcp's are most convenient and readily available form. Ensure there are no contraindications to their use.
  - Cyclic estrogen/progesterone may be an option.

- Avoid use of Depo-Provera, as BC in at risk athletes (thin endurance athletes or gymnasts).

18.2 Osteoporosis

J Am Acad Orthop Sug 1998;6:349

Cause: In the athlete is usually due to long-standing estrogen deficiency (EAA).

Epidem:
- Occurs in athletes in association with amenorrhea. Most common in long distance runners, triathletes, gymnasts, ballet dancers, etc.
- >1.3 million fractures per yr attributable to osteoporosis in the general population.

Pathophys: Estrogen responsible for stimulating normal osteoblastic cell function in replacing matrix. Chronic low estrogen states lead to gradual loss of bone mass with normal ratio of mineral to osteoid matrix.
- In EAA, 4% trabecular bone loss in first 12 mo, 10% per yr after this.

Sx: None in early stages; symptoms of bone injury (stress fractures, acute fractures) in later stages.

Si:
- None in early stages.
- "Dowager's hump" (thoracic kyphosis) in later stages.
- Acute or stress fractures.

X-ray:

Heel ultrasound: Relatively inexpensive, yet fairly sensitive screening test.

Dual energy x-ray absorptiometry (DEXA) scan: Detect early bone loss and report values relative to an age adjusted mean. Currently becoming widely available. Recommended to have base line tested on all amenorrheic athletes.

ISSUES UNIQUE TO THE FEMALE ATHLETE

Lab: Evaluation as outlined for EAA (see 18.1); calcium and phosphorus levels are normal.

Crs: Bone loss does not fully recover if estrogen deficiency continues longer than 24-36 mo.

Rx: Prevention is most effective treatment. All female athletes should be queried regarding menstrual history. W delayed menarche or secondary amenorrhea, further evaluation and treatment with estrogen replacement should be undertaken; w established osteoporosis, aggressive management recommended.
- Calcium supplements: 1200 mg/d as calcium carbonate (eg, Tums, Caltrate, Oscal) or calcium citrate (Citraca). Vitamin D, 400 to 800 U/d, should be taken with calcium.
- For severe osteoporosis additional nonhormonal medical treatment may be added. Examples include: Alendronate (Fosamax) 5 mg po qam, Calcitonin (Miacalcin nasal spray 200 U/d, or injectable calcitonin, 50 to 100 U/d) or Raloxifene (Evista, 60 mg po qd) a selective estrogen receptor modulator.

18.3 Eating Disorders

Clin Sports Med 2000;19:199

Epidem:
- Effects up to 20% of adolescent and young adult females.
- Most common in endurance sports (running, XC skiing), performance sports (ballet, gymnastics, figure skating), and wt class sports (wrestling, boxing).

Pathophys: These are psychologic conditions, which lead to significant endocrinologic disorders. DSM-IV describes two main eating disorders which are common in the athletic population:
1. Anorexia nervosa, characterized by:
   - Refusal to maintain a minimal normal wt.
   - Intense fear of gaining wt.

- Disturbance in the interpretation of body image (lack of insight into eating disorder).
- Amenorrhea (in postmenarchal females, failure to menstruate for 3 consecutive mo).
- Classified as restrictive type (failure to consume adequate calories) and purging type (consume adequate calories but purge after eating).
2. Bulimia, characterized by:
   - Recurrent episodes of uncontrolled binge eating.
   - Recurrent inappropriate compensatory purging.
   - Occurring at least 2 × per wk for 3 mo.
   - Self-evaluation is unduly based on body size and shape.
   - The disturbance does not occur exclusively with episodes of anorexia nervosa.
   - Classified as purging type (vomiting, diuretics, laxative use), and nonpurging (compensate with fasting or exercise).

Sx:

- A very high index of suspicion is required, as the athlete will rarely present with a chief complaint of "eating disorder."
- May seek care due to fatigue or performance decrement. May have associated musculoskeletal complaints (eg, stress reactions or fractures).
- Frequently is brought to physician's attention by athletic trainer, coach, parent, or teammates.
- Amenorrhea.

Si:

- Below ideal body wt, typically with a low percent body fat.
- Dental disease due to gastric acid effects on teeth and gums (tooth discoloration, caries, gingivitis).
- Russell's sign: discoloration of one (or more) fingers due to acid effects when inducing vomiting.
- Parotid or other salivary gland enlargement.

Lab: Nutritional workup including: CBC, prealbumin.

Crs: Typically requires long-term therapy, relapses common, death does occur.

Rx:

- Aggressive treatment initiated immediately upon making the diagnosis. Should involve physician, psychologist, nutritionist, coach, parents (if appropriate), and athlete.
- Set target wt at IBW for height, age, and sport.
- Selective serotonin reuptake inhibiting (SSRI) medications are generally useful in treatment.
- Amenorrhea should be evaluated and treated as outlined in previous section.
- Restrict training until IBW is attained and must be maintained to continue training/competition.
- Athlete, coach, parent, and team education is crucial for long-term success.
- Psychologic care is typically needed for extended period.
- Should consider inpatient management if weight falls below 70-75% IBW.

18.4 Exercise in Pregnancy

ACOG Technical Bulletin 1994 No 189, Washington, DC; J Reprod Med 2005;50:181

Physiologic Changes:

- Cardiovascular: increased blood volume, cardiac output, pulse, decreased peripheral vascular resistance.
- Respiratory: minute ventilation increases 50%; 10-20% increase in basal oxygen requirements.
- Metabolic requirements: increased basal metabolic rate approx 300 kcal/d.

- Musculoskeletal: hormonal effects on joint laxity. Altered center of gravity due to uterine and breast enlargement.

Scientific Basis:

- Previous recommendations were very conservative, and possibly detrimental to health of mother and fetus as a result.
- Recommendations have not previously been based on scientific study.
- Few scientific studies on outcome have been done.
- Current recommendations based on known physiologic changes, limited studies, and case reports.
- Generally felt that light to moderate exercise is safe and beneficial with certain exceptions (see below).

Benefits of Exercise:

- Fetal well-being: decreased incidence of meconium births, cord entanglements, and abnormal fetal tracings. Higher APGAR scores.
- Pregnancy outcome: no increase in spontaneous abortions, congenital abnormalities, or placental abnormalities.
- Pregnancy duration: slight shortening of overall length of gestation.
- Labor: shortens first and second stages of labor.
- Maternal well-being: decreased pain and discomfort, decreased wt gain, improved fitness.

Contraindications:

- Premature rupture of membranes.
- Preterm labor.
- Vaginal bleeding, placenta previa, abruptio placentae.
- Fetal distress, growth retardation.
- Preeclampsia.
- Renal disease, heart disease.
- Multiple pregnancy (>twins).

Relative Contraindications:

- Uncontrolled hypertension.
- Moderate to severe anemia.
- Poorly controlled diabetes.
- Excessively high or low wt (gain).
- Smoking or excessive alcohol abuse.
- Twins after the second trimester.
- Previous sedentary lifestyle.
- Pulmonary disease, cardiac dysrythmia, mild to moderate valvular disease.

Exercise Recommendations in Pregnancy:

- Individualize based on previous activity, health during pregnancy, fetal well-being, and contraindications (as listed above).
- Exercise should be light to moderate in intensity performed at least 3 × per wk.
- Avoid exercise in a supine position, which will diminish cardiac output w specific reduction in uterine blood flow.
- Because of diminished functional lung volume, oxygen availability will be diminished. Important that the women avoid activity to a level that leads to excessive dyspnea.
- Take into account changing abilities as pregnancy progresses. Substantial changes in size, wt, center of gravity increase risk of falls in many activities. Avoid activities with a risk of falling or abdominal trauma.

Chapter 19

Gastrointestinal Problems

19.1 General Epidemiology

N Z Med 1994;107:328, Am J Gastroenterol 1999;94:1570

- gi symptoms most often reported include gastroesophageal (GE) reflux, abdominal pain, diarrhea, and nausea.
- Incidence greater than 80% in certain groups of running athletes.
- Rowers, cross-country skiers, swimmers and cyclists, report similar problems.
- Runners have a higher incidence of lower gi symptoms vs upper gi symptoms (71% vs 36% respectively).
- Cyclists had a fairly even split between upper and lower gi symptoms (67% vs 64% respectively).

19.2 Upper GI Symptoms

Curr Sports Med Rep 2004;3:107; Aust J Sci Med Sport 1996;28:93; Ann IM 1990;112:429

Causes/Pathophys:
- Transient relaxation of the lower esophageal sphincter (LES) due to air swallowing, alcohol, caffeine, high-fat foods, smoking, and many drugs.
- Increase in acid production has been suggested; however, recent studies indicate that decreased gastric mucosal secretion, resulting from reduced splanchnic blood flow, is more likely.

- Accentuated by NSAID use, emotional stress, or any factor that increases acid production.
- Delayed gastric emptying, seen w strenuous exercise, may also contribute.
- *Helicobacter pylori* infection should be considered in cases of chronic or recurrent upper gi symptoms.

Sx:

- Common upper gi symptoms include belching, nausea, vomiting, and epigastric pain.
- Usually experienced during maximal exertion.
- May mimic symptoms of cardiac disease.
- Symptoms are generally worse w increasing intensity or prolonged duration of exercise and are more severe with immediate postprandial exercise (within 3 hr of eating).
- Documentation of training habits, NSAID use, diet, and prior history (or family history) of gastritis, peptic ulcer disease, inflammatory bowel disease, or other gi problems important.

Si: Generally nonspecific, may be epigastric tenderness.

Crs: Usually effectively treated.

Lab:

- Complete blood cell count to assess hemoglobin and hematocrit to ensure that there is no significant blood loss.
- Liver function testing with transaminases, bilirubin, and amylase are relatively inexpensive and will help to exclude other causes of upper gi symptoms such as hepatitis, pancreatitis, and biliary tract disease.
- Serologic testing for *H. pylori* is now available and is indicated in the runner with chronic dyspepsia.

Other testing: Care must be taken to rule out more serious causes of epigastric pain, most importantly those of a cardiac etiology.

- An electrocardiogram (EKG) or electrocardiographic stress test should be obtained in athletes presenting with epigastric pain and associated cardiac risk factors (> 40 y/o, smoking history, family history, hyperlipidemia or comorbid disease state) or if associated symptoms suggest cardiac origin (shortness of breath, diaphoresis, radiating pain).

- Endoscopy (EGD) should be performed in pts w recurrent or persistent symptoms in the face of treatment.
- Ambulatory pH monitoring and LES manometry is considered w refractory symptoms following an otherwise normal evaluation.

Rx: Should be approached stepwise as the evaluation proceeds

- Most often, simple changes in diet, meal timing, and training habits will alleviate these symptoms.
  - Avoiding large meals 2-3 hr prior to training and high concentration (hyperosmolar) feeds while training may prevent symptoms.
  - The use of low-fat, low-protein, liquid calorie and electrolyte solutions is an effective means of supplying immediate pre-exercise calories while minimizing GE reflux.
  - Isotonic fluids tend to cause fewer upper gi symptoms and are the best source for calorie replacement while exercising.
- Athletes may also reduce these symptoms by temporarily decreasing training or by alternating running with a lower-impact workout, eg, cycling or swimming.
- Medical therapy options include:
  - Antacids (aluminum hydroxide and magnesium salts) are useful in the treatment of mild symptoms. These should be taken immediately before beginning exercise and can be repeated during the workout, as needed.
  - H_2 receptor blockers (ranitidine, 150 mg bid, famotidine, 20 mg per d, and cimetidine, 400 mg $2 \times$ qd), have been shown to be effective in decreasing upper gi symptoms in runners.
  - The gastric proton pump inhibitors (omeprazole, 20 mg qd, lansoprazole, 15 mg qd), are very effective in treating GERD but have not been studied specifically in athletes.

- Prokinetic agents, metoclopramide (Reglan), 10 mg 1 hr prior to running reduce GE reflux by reducing transit time in the upper GI tract. These medications have undesired side effects in comparison to the other choices.
- Discontinuation of NSAIDs or the substitution of these medications w a COX-2 selective anti-inflammatory (Celebrex, 200 mg qd, Vioxx 25 mg qd) is usually prudent.

19.3 Lower GI Symptoms

Jama 1980;243:1743; Ann IM 1984;100:843; Int J Sports Med 1989;10:suppl22

Epidem: 37-54% of runners experience bowel urgency either during or immediately following a strenuous workout.

Cause/Pathophys: The precise physiology of runner's diarrhea is not well understood, although a number of etiologies have been suggested:
- Rapid shifts in intestinal fluid and electrolytes with strenuous exercise results in colonic irritability and cramping.
- Increased parasympathetic tone seen w moderate exercise causes increased peristalsis leading to rapid bowel transit and cramping.
- In more strenuous exercise, sympathetic nervous system stimulation increases the release of gastroenteropancreatic hormones (gastrin, motilin, and endogenous opioids).
- Ischemic enteropathy and gi bleeding may also cause runner's diarrhea (see sx).
- Infectious etiologies should also be considered in acute diarrheal illnesses in runners.

    In severe cases, runner's diarrhea may result in significant dehydration and has been implicated in the development of rhabdomyolysis and acute tubular necrosis.

Sx: Lower gi symptoms include fecal urgency, loose stools, and frank diarrhea; these symptoms are usually precipitated w increasing training mileage or with particularly intensive workouts. Frequently the athlete is forced to interrupt the workout as a result of these symptoms. A careful history including:

- Symptom character and severity including the presence of diarrhea, melena, hematochezia, or hematemesis and association w exercise, meals, or other stresses.
- Any recent changes in training intensity, duration, or distance, should be quantified.
- NSAID use, history of recent travel, and preexisting illness are also important etiologic factors.
- A history or family history of inflammatory bowel disease, gastritis, peptic ulcer disease, and other causes of gi bleeding.

Si:

- Typically nonspecific.
- Mild abdominal tenderness common.
- Palpate to ensure no hepatomegally.
- Digital rectal exam heme content determination.

Lab:

- Stool evaluation for fecal heme content, leukocytes, ovum and parasites, and stool cultures, to determine the presence of inflammatory or infectious etiologies.
- A complete blood cell count should be done to evaluate for possible anemia.

Other testing: Further workup may include endoscopy or radiography for chronic symptoms (see discussion under gi blood loss).

Rx:

- Reduction in training intensity or distance for 1-2 wk w a gradual return to the previous high-intensity workouts.
- Exercise substitution and cross training w low-impact (non-running) activities also help to reduce the symptoms, while allowing the athlete to maintain cardiovascular fitness.

- Dietary manipulations may be of some use in the prevention of lower gi symptoms. A complete liquid diet on the day prior to a long-distance competition or planned strenuous workout may decrease symptoms during the event.
- Low-residue (low-fiber) diet may be helpful in some athletes.
- Antidiarrhea medications should be used w caution due to potential side effects. Antispasmodics such as loperimide (4 mg initially, then 2 mg as needed to 16 mg/d) are usually safe. Anticholinergic medications (Lomotil or Motofen) should be avoided as they can affect sweating w increased risk of heat injury.

19.4 Gastrointestinal Blood Loss

Phy Sportsmed 1990;18:75; Aust J Sci Med Sport 1995;27:3; Gut 1987;28:896

Epidem:
- Review of studies suggests that the gi bleeding may be distance- or effort-related (dose-dependent).
- 20% incidence of occult blood in the stools of runners completing a marathon; w up to 6% reporting frank hematochezia.
- 87% pos conversion rate on stool occult blood testing in runners following an ultra-distance running event.

Cause/Pathophys: Several possible mechanisms for gastrointestinal bleeding in runners have been suggested:
- Running induced ischemic enteropathy. Splanchnic blood flow is reduced by approximately 70%-80% of normal w strenuous cardiovascular exercise. When low blood flow is maintained for a long period, it can lead to local tissue ischemia, necrosis, and superficial mucosal erosions, resulting in intraluminal bleeding.

- By a similar mechanism, reduced gi blood flow also contributes to the development of hemorrhagic gastritis, which is associated with gi blood loss in long-distance runners.
- Another theory involves mechanical trauma to the bowel similar to that described in other hollow viscera, such as the bladder and ureters. The repetitive jarring of the intestines results in serosal and mucosal injury.
- Hemorrhagic gastritis may result from mechanical stress via traction forces of the diaphragm and gastrophrenic ligaments on the gastric fundus.
- The relationship between nonsteroidal anti-inflammatory drug (NSAID) use and gi blood loss is not clear. NSAIDs have been associated w the development of gastritis and peptic ulcer disease; however, the studies on gi blood loss in the athlete have not shown any direct correlation.
- Perianal disease, including hemorrhoids, fissures, and perianal chafing, is another possible cause of gi blood loss in athletes.

Sx: Athletes report bloody diarrhea, melanic stools, or hematochezia.

Si: Heme-pos stool sampling on DRE; otherwise nonspecific.

Lab: Initial evaluation as above for runner's diarrhea.

X-ray:
- Barium enema rarely useful.
- Flexible sigmoidoscopy, colonoscopy, and esophagogastroduodenoscopy (EGD) to determine the focus of blood loss.

Rx:
- Short-term reduction in training along w exercise substitution (discussed in 19.3).
- In cases related to hemorrhagic gastritis, the use of H_2 antagonist agents, (ranitidine, 150 mg 2 × qd, famotidine, 20 mg qd, or cimetidine, 400 mg 2 × qd) is very effective over the course of several d.

- In endurance athletes who are predisposed to upper gi blood loss (ultra-distance runners or previous history of UGI blood loss), pre-race treatment with H_2 antagonists is effective in preventing blood loss.
- Discontinuation of NSAIDs or substitution with a COX-2 selective medication (Celebrex, 200 mg qd, and Vioxx 25 mg qd) should be advised in most cases of bloody diarrhea.

19.5 Hepatic Injury: Abnormal Liver Function Tests (LFTs)

Mayo Clin Proc 1980;55:113; Med Sci Sports Exerc 1995;27:1590; Int J Sports Med 1990;11:441

Cause: Results from ischemic insult due to decreased oxygen tension in the hepatic blood supply.

Epidem: Liver enzyme elevations are most affected by long-distance running.

Pathophys: The damage to the liver is readily reversible when exercise is stopped, w enzyme levels usually returning to normal within 1 wk.

Sx: Asymptomatic.

Si: Usually normal PE.

Lab:
- Increased serum glutamic-oxaloacetic transaminase (SGOT), alanine aminotransferase (ALT), creatine kinase, aspartate aminotransferase (AST), bilirubin, alkaline phosphatase, creatinine phosphatase, and lactic dehydrogenase (LDH) have all been described in runners. While these can indicate liver injury, they may also be related to musculoskeletal trauma.
- More specific indicators of hepatocellular injury, glutamate dehydrogenase (GLDH) and gamma-glutamyl-transferase (GGT) have been found to be elevated in long-distance runners.

- The gradual serum reductions of albumin seen in ultra-distance runners further support the possibility of hepatic injury in these athletes.

X-ray: None indicated.

Rx: While there is no evidence that these exercise-related enzyme elevations lead to long-term sequelae, it would seem prudent to limit exercise until LFTs normalize.

19.6 Abdominal Pain (The "Side Stitch")

Med Sci Sports Exerc 1995;27:623; Phy Sportsmed 1985;13:187

Epidem: The most common cause of abdominal pain with exercise; affects runners, trained and untrained, as they significantly increase their mileage and in untrained persons initiating an exercise program.

Cause/Pathophys:
- The precise etiology is not known, but most likely due to diaphragmatic muscle spasm related to hypoxia.
- Other possible explanations include hepatic capsule irritation, pleural irritation, abdominal adhesions, and right colonic gas pains.
- These pains are often worse w postprandial exercise.

Sx: Described as an aching sensation during exercise in the right upper abdominal quadrant.

Si: Nonspecific with classic "stitch"; abdominal tenderness or constitutional symptoms may indicate more significant diagnosis (see below).

Crs: Generally resolves w improved conditioning.

Lab/X-ray: None indicated.

Rx:

- Pt may get some relief by stretching the right arm over the head or by forced expiration against pursed lips.
- Stopping exercise nearly always results in immediate cessation of symptoms.
- The frequency and severity of stitches usually decrease as the overall fitness of the athlete improves.
- Exclude other causes of abdominal pain (omental infarction, bowel infarction, and hepatic vein thrombosis), which typically present w significant illness:
  - These are very rare events and are generally accompanied by unremitting pain, severe systemic illness, collapse, and multisystem failure.
  - Most common after long-distance competition and require emergent surgical intervention.

Chapter 20

Infectious Disease

20.1 Acute Febrile Illness

Phy Sportsmed 1996;24:44; Phy Sportsmed 1999;27:47; The Team Physician Handbook. 2nd ed. St. Louis: Mosby 1997;225

Cause: Viral or bacterial causes.

Pathophys: Change in hypothalamic set point to aid in fighting infection; physiologic response includes increased sensible fluid loss, increased resting heart rate, increased basal metabolism, decreased pulmonary gas diffusion, decreased concentration, increased susceptibility to heat illness and injury.

Sx: May or may not be associated with myalgia, pulmonary, upper respiratory, gi, or GU symptoms.

Si: Temp >100.4°; focal or nonfocal signs.

Crs: Usually self-limiting.

Cmplc: Untreated focal infection; sudden death due to myocarditis, infecting fellow competitors.

Diff Dx: Early focal infection (UTI, pyelonephrites, pneumonia, pharyngitis, sinusitis, gastroenteritis), CVD.

Lab: Usually not indicated except for UTI or more severe infections.

Rx:
- Acetaminophen (Tylenol) 650-1000 mg qid.
- Ibuprofen (Motrin) 400 mg qid to 800 mg tid; beware of gi and renal effects.

- Preventing the spread of infection (Phy Sportsmed 2003;31:23):
  - Limit exposure (restrict ill athletes).
  - Handwashing and daily showering.
  - Protect skin (eg, change socks, take care of blisters and abrasions).
  - Safeguard water source: safe, clean drinking water; care and cleanliness of water containers; do not share water bottle.
  - Clean practice surfaces and uniforms; mat and court care.
  - Protect individual immunity: avoid overtraining; slow down when inappropriately fatigued; pay attention to nutrition, hydration, and sleep; immunizations (Td and *H. flu*; Hep A and Hep B).
  - Be prepared for universal precautions to protect from hand and body fluids: use gloves, disposal bags, careful handling of sharps, antiseptic soaps, and cleansers.

Return to Activity:
- "Neck check" (Phy Sportsmed 1993;21:125):
  - Resolution of below-the-neck symptoms (fever, severe cough, diarrhea/vomiting, myalgias).
  - Normal hydration.
  - Beware postviral bronchial reactivity—may need bronchodilator (Phy Sportsmed 1993;21:125).
- Generally 2 d rest for every d of lost training.
- Begin training at 50% intensity and if feeling OK after 5-10 min, train at full intensity.
- If recovering from URI, SI or OM nl Valsalva function for altitude and aquatic sports.
- If there is a TM perforation, it should be resolved before altitude or aquatic sports.

20.2 Infectious Mononucleosis (IM)

Clin Sports Med 2004;23:485; Am Fam Phys 2004;70:1279; Phy
    Sportsmed 2002;30:27; Phy Sportsmed 1996;24:49; Clin Sports
    Med 1997;16:635

Cause: Epstein-Barr virus of the herpes family.

Epidem:
- 95% infected by 25 y/o; highest prevalence in 15-25 y/o age
  group, but only 50% are symptomatic.
- Affects 25% of college-aged individuals.
- Not highly contagious among college roommates.

Pathophys: Infects B cells; transmitted by intimate contact.

Sx: Fever, fatigue, sore throat, ± abdominal pain; possible exposure
    history to IM.

Si: Tired-appearing; purulent pharyngitis; diffuse adenopathy (esp pos-
    terior cervical), signs of hepatosplenomegaly.

Crs: Usually self-limiting, but may have prolonged fatigue.

Cmplc: Loss of training time, school or work performance due to pro-
    longed fatigue; upper airway obstruction; splenic rupture;
    Guillain-Barré; thrombocytopenia; or hemolytic anemia.

Diff Dx: GABS, CMV, enterovirus, coxsackie, GC, mycoplasma.

Lab: Mild leukocytosis with increased ATL count; elevated transami-
    nases; elevated urine specific gravity or BUN if dehydrated; may
    have hemolytic anemia or thrombocytopenia; throat culture or
    rapid strep test.

X-ray: Consider US, CT, or MRI to eval splenomegaly in large ath-
    letes (hard to examine or those requesting early return to activ-
    ity); spleen longitudinal length <15 cm or spleen to ipsilateral
    kidney ratio <1.25 (Pediatr Radiol 1998;28:98).

INFECTIOUS DISEASE

Rx:

- Symptomatic management of fever and fatigue.
- No contact activity for minimum of 3 wk, usually 4-6 wk.
- Low-impact aerobics as tolerated over first 2-4 wk.
- Appropriate antibiotics for strep pharyngitis (penicillin or erythromycin).
- Corticosteroids for significant tonsilar enlargement or elevated transaminases.
- Referral for splenic rupture; airway compromise; hemolytic anemia or thrombocytopenia; consider referral of those placed on oral corticosteroids.

Return to Activity: Resolved constitutional symptoms and adequate energy level; nl labs (CBC and LFTs); normal physical exam; neg imaging study if indicated (see X-ray).

20.3 Diarrhea

Phy Sportsmed 1997;25:80; Clin Sports Med 1997;16:635; Gastroenterol Clin No Amer 2003;32:1249

Cause: Infection, medications, inflammatory.

Epidem: Viral (Rotavirus, Norwalk agent, enteroviruses); bacterial (Shigella, Salmonella, Yersinia); protozoan (Giardia, E. histolytica).

Pathophys: Increased water content of stool.

Sx: Fever, myalgia, diarrhea (watery/bloody); h/o travel.

Si: Fever, signs of dehydration, ± abdominal pain.

Crs: Usually self-limiting.

Cmplc: Dehydration and electrolyte dysfunction; heat illness or other injury if training intensity while ill; sepsis; contagiousness.

Diff Dx: IBD, IBS, diverticulitis, diverticulosis, cancer, ischemic bowel.

Lab: Fecal WBC, stool culture, consider CBC and chemistries, if signs of dehydration or severe infection.

X-ray: AAS for signs of significant illness.

Rx:
- Fluids (oral or iv).
- Antispasmodics.
  - Dicyclomine (Bentyl) 10-20 mg qid.
  - Phenobarbital/atropine/hyoscyamine (Donatal) 1-2 tab qid.
- Loperamide (Imodium) 4 mg initial, followed by 2 mg prn loose stool to max 16 mg/d.
- Antibiotics for pos cultures or for traveler's diarrhea, if in foreign country (Cipro 500 mg/d for 5 d).
- Avoid caffeine, NSAIDs, and high carbohydrate drinks/foods.

Return to Activity: Guided by hydration state, risk of infecting others, and desire to return.

Skin Infections of Concern in Contact Sports

20.4 Cellulitis

Clin Sports Med 2004;23:473; Phy Sportsmed 1997;25:45

Cause: *Streptococcus, S. aureus.*

Epidem: Common in all contact sports (esp wrestling, judo, karate).

Pathophys: Local soft tissue trauma (abrasion, friction blister, arthropod/human/animal bite) causing epidermal breakdown and secondary bacterial invasion into subcutaneous tissues.

Sx: Fever, local soft tissue pain, swelling, and possible drainage.

Si: Local area of skin breakdown (abrasion, excoriation, blister or other), erythema, heat, induration, lymphangitic streaking.

Cmplc: Sepsis, endocarditis, osteomyelitis.

Diff Dx: Venous stasis, if on LE; myositis; muscle contusion/hematoma.

Lab: Elevated WBC.

X-ray: Consider soft tissue film to look for gas in severe cases.

Rx:
- Warm compress, elevation, antipyretics, and analgesics.
- Antistaphylococcal antibiotics:
  - Amoxicillin/clavulanate (Augmentin) 875 mg bid.
  - Dicloxacillin 250-500 mg qid.
  - Cephalexin (Keflex) 250-500 mg qid.
  - Levofloxin 250-500 mg qd.
  - Ciprofloxacin 250-750 mg bid.

Return to Activity: Dry or clinically resolved; resolved constitutional symptoms.

20.5 Herpes Gladiatorum

Phy Sportsmed 2004;32:23; Phy Sportsmed 1997;25:45; Curr Sports Med Rep 2004;3:277; Am J Sports Med 2003;5:309; Clin Sports Med 1997;16:635

Cause: HSV I or II.

Epidem: By age 50 90% of population is HSV-I seropositive; estimated prevalence in one wrestling season of 2.6% for HS and 7.6% for college.

Pathophys: Primary infections for close contact with infectious athletes or from wrestling/gymnastic mats; may have recurrent outbreaks from prior infection.

Sx: Skin eruption w antecedent burning pain; low-grade fever; myalgia.

Si: Clusters of vesicles on erythematous base that may occur anywhere (face, neck, trunk).

Crs: Left untreated spontaneous resolution will occur in 7-10 d.

Cmplc: Recurrent infection, contamination of sport equipment and spread of infection to others, secondary infection, scarring, neuralgia.

Diff Dx: Abscess, eczema, or contact dermatitis.

Lab: Tzanck prep demonstrating multinucleated giant cells; viral culture of base of vesicle.

Rx:

- Analgesics.
- Astringents (topical Domeboro compresses).
- Oral antivirals.
  - Acyclovir (Zovirax) 400 mg tid for 5-7 d.
  - Valacyclovir (Valtrex) 500 mg bid for 5 d.
  - Famciclovir (Famvir) 125 mg bid for 5 d.

Return to Activity: No new vesicles and old vesicles dry and well-crested, resolved erythema, no secondary infection; for recurrent case, consider prophylaxis with Valtrex 1 gm/d (Am J Med Sports 2003;5:309) or Valtrex 500 mg bid or Acyclovir 400 mg bid (Phy Sportsmed 2004;32:23).

20.6 Tinea Gladiatorum (Ringworm)

Clin J Sp Med 2002;12:165; Phy Sportsmed 2004;32:23; Phy Sportsmed 1997;25:45; Clin Sports Med 1997;16:635

Cause: Dermatophytes usually from Trichophyton genus.

Epidem: Of concern in close contact sports (wrestling and martial arts); in a recent study in PA, 84% of wrestling teams had at least 1 wrestler out at any time with ringworm (Clin J Sp Med 2002;12:165).

Pathophys: Moisture and direct skin contact with infected mat or athletic equipment and abrasions, allowing local infection.

Sx: Pruritic, slowly enlarging rash.

Si: Discoid, red, raised patch, with some scale and/or crust.

Crs: Self-limiting; slow growth; no long-term sequelae.

Cmplc: Secondary infection, spread of disease to others.

Diff Dx: Contact dermatitis, abrasion, psoriasis, seborrheic dermatitis.

Lab: Exam of scrapings under KOH demonstrating branching hyphae.

Rx:

Topical antifungals:
- Clotrimazole 1% (Lotrimin) bid or tid.
- Terbinafine (Lamisil) qd.
- Econazole (Spectazole) qd or bid.
- Ketoconazole (Nizoril) 2% cream qd.

Oral antifungals (for refractory or recurrent cases):
- Ketoconazole (Nizoral) 200-400 mg qd for 4 wk.
- Itraconazole 200 mg qd for 2 wk.
- Terbinafine (Lamisil) 250 mg qd for 2 wk.
- Fluconazole 150 mg 1 ×/wk for 1-4 wk.

Return to Activity: 72 hrs of therapy may be covered; when lesion is flattened and scaling resolved; consider prophylaxis for recurrent cases with fluconazole 150 mg 1 ×/wk.

Chapter 21

Other Medical Problems

21.1 Overtraining (Staleness)

Phy Sportsmed 2003;31:25; Phy Sportsmed 2001;29:35; Med Sci
Sports Exerc 1997;30:1173; Med Sci Sports Exerc 1998;30:1146;
Sports Med 1998;30:1140; Sports Med 2000;32:317; Sports Med
1996;21:80; Sports Med 1998;26:1; Sports Med 1998;26:177;
Sports Med 1999;27:73; J Sport Sci 1997;15:341

Cause: Excessive training and competition without adequate recovery.

Epidem: Affects 5-15% of elite athletes at any one time.

Pathophys:

Definitions:
- Overreaching-acute phase of increased training load w short-
  term deterioration in performance (usually <2 wk).
- Overtraining-maladaptive response to an extended period of
  training overload w inability to recover within 2-wk rest
  period.

Multiple hypotheses:
- Chronic glycogen depletion: chronic nutritional deficiency
  leading to chronic glycogen depletion and increased oxidation
  of branched chain amino acids and a change in the BCAA:
  free try ratio and ultimately central fatigue (Med Sci Sports
  Exerc 1998;30:1146).
- Autonomic imbalance: increased sympathetic activity from
  stress and overloaded target organs and increased catabolism

leading to decreased sympathetic intrinsic activity (Med Sci Sports Exerc 1998;30:1140).

- Central fatigue hypothesis: peripheral fatigue and nutrient depletion leading to the consumption of BCAA with subsequent change in the BCAA: free try ratio; with elevated CNS free try leading to elevated CNS 5HT and central fatigue (Med Sci Sports Exerc 1997;30:1173).
- Glutamine hypothesis (immune dysfunction): overload training leading to depressed glutamine production from muscle tissue; glutamine deficiency, as well as acute exercise stress on the immune system create immunologic open window, leading to repeated minor infections and systemic stress (Sports Med 1998;26:177).
- Cytokine hypothesis: incomplete recovery of locally damaged tissues with overload causing a local inflammatory response to become systemic with elevated pro-inflammatory cytokines IL-1β, TNF-α, and IL-6 (Med Sci Sports Exerc 2000;32:317; Med Sci Sports Exerc 2004;36:794).

Fatigue

Physiologic fatigue:
- Insufficient sleep, nutritional disorder, jet lag, pregnancy, excessive competition, overreaching.

Pathologic fatigue:
- Medical disorders, mood disorders, chronic fatigue syndrome, overtraining.

Sx: Fatigue; decreased performance; overuse injuries (musculoskeletal manifestation of overtraining); sleep disturbance; mood disorder.

Si: Elevated resting HR (usually >10 BPM over baseline) (Clin J Sp Med 2000;10:279); decreased LBM; depressed mood on various evaluation tools; otherwise essentially normal exam.

Crs: Depends on duration and severity of symptoms and the athletes and coaches management.

Cmplc: Early retirement, poor performance during key periods (Olympics, etc), injury.

Diff Dx:
- Infectious disease: infectious mono, Lymes, pneumonia, CMV, other viral inf (see 20.1 and 20.2).
- Metabolic disorders: anemia, diabetes, hypo- or hyperthyroid.
- Substance abuse: ETOH, cocaine, marijuana, stimulants.
- Mood disorder: depression, BPD, other.
- Cancer: lymphoma, leukemia, other.
- Pregnancy.

Lab: W initial visit consider CBC, ESR, Chem 20, TSH, ferritin, serum β-HCG, monospot; at f/u consider urine drug screen or other labs based on history and examination.

Rx:
- Rest (initially for 2 wk); if recovered, then resume more balanced training.
- More significant symptoms may require longer periods of rest from training and competition.
- Upon return to activity need more balanced training (periodization) w periods of relative rest and cross training to avoid monotony and overuse w careful attention to sleep, nutrition, hydration, social support, and stretching.

Return to Activity: Monitor overall recovery process and listen to the body's signals (mood, myalgias, sense of well-being).

21.2 Exertional Rhabdomyolysis

Arch IM 1976;136:692; Mil Med 1996;161:564; Am Fam Phys 2002;65:907; Am Fam Phys 1995;52:502; Phy Sportsmed 2004;32:15; Phy Sportsmed 2002;30:37

Cause: Muscle breakdown from severe, exhaustive exercise.

Epidem:

- Many reports associated with mass training or mass participation, as in military training or police training of recruits.
- Risk factors of high ambient temp and high humidity, poor conditioning, dehydration, compromised nutritional state, hypoxia, sickle cell disease or trait, medication use (aspirin, phenothiazines, anticholinergics), drugs (cocaine, alcohol), renal insufficiency, recent viral illness, or prior heat injury.
- Recent reports of exertional rhabdomyolysis associated with creatine supplementation (J Am Board Fam Prac 2000;13:134).

Pathophys: Severe muscle breakdown with release of toxins and electrolytes leading to hypernatremia, hyperkalemia, hyperuricemia, lactic acidosis, and secondary oliguric renal failure.

Sx: H/o exhaustive exercise session (often eccentric type); delayed onset muscle soreness with local swelling; dark urine.

Si: Significant local compartment soft tissue swelling; pain with passive motion of muscles; decreased urine output; may have signs of multiorgan failure or even collapse.

Crs: Variable depending on extend of muscle damage and comorbid disease.

Cmplc: Renal failure (more associated with CPKs >16,000 (Am Fam Phys 2002;65:907), multiorgan failure, acute compartment syndrome, ARDS, DIC.

Diff Dx: Delayed onset muscle soreness, exertional compartment syndrome without rhabdomyolysis, consider workup for metabolic myopathy (impaired muscle metabolism or inherited enzyme deficiency) for recurrent cases (Phy Sportsmed 2002;30:37).

Lab: Elevated CPK (absolute number is not diagnostic, but a value >3000 is considered to be pos), urine myoglobin (or pos dipstick for blood without RBC on micro), elevated LFTs, BUN, creat, sodium, potassium and lactic acidosis; secondary hypocalcemia, hyperphosphatemia, hypoalbuminemia and oliguria with subse-

quent DIC (dec fibrinogen and Plt and inc FSP, coags); muscle
biopsy is needed to diagnose metabolic myopathies.

Rx:
- Aggressive fluid resuscitation (4-10 L in first 24 hrs) to maintain urine output of 300 cc/hr until myoglobinuria resolved (Am Fam Phys 2002;65:905).
- Lasix 40-120 mg.
- Mannitol (100 cc of 25% solution).
- Consider alkalization of urine.
- Monitor and manage compartment syndrome with fasciotomy, as required.
- Monitor electrolytes and treat deficient or excess states, as indicated (potassium, calcium).
- In severe cases of renal failure consider dialysis.

Return to Activity: May take several mo up to 1 yr; begin with stretching and low-impact aerobics, then concentric exercise and slow advancement as tolerated, maintaining adequate nutrition and hydration during recovery exercise.

21.3 Exertional Hyponatremia

GSSI 2003;16:1; Nejm 2005;352:1550; Nejm 2000;342:1581; Am Fam Phys 2004;69:2387; Mil Med 2002;167:432; Curr Sports Med Rep 2002;4:197

Cause: Excessive fluid intake, inappropriate secretion of arginine vasopressin (AVP) or SIADH.

Epidem: More commonly seen in endurance events in particular marathons; as much as 17% of marathon runners; more common in women, slower runners (odds ratio of 4:1 for run times of 5 hr); extremes of BMI and pre-race NSAID use (Nejm 2005;352:1550).

Pathophys: Inappropriate AVP (ADH) secretion despite hypo-osmolar state; likely related to stress cytokines (IL-6).

Sx: Headache, nausea, vomiting, cramps, lethargy, disorientation, seizure, coma.

Si: Exertional collapse with normal temperature, wt gain during race, ataxia.

Crs: Variable depending on severity and recognition and proper management.

Cmplc: Seizure, coma, death.

Diff Dx: Exertional collapse, (see 17.1) muscle cramps, heat exhaustion/stroke (see 2.8), exertional rhabdomyolysis (see 21.2).

Lab: Serum sodium (<125 mmol/L severe, 126-130 moderate, 131-135 mild).

X-ray: N/a.

Rx:

- For severe cases consider starting 3% hypertonic saline at 100 cc/hr, monitoring Na every 1-2 hrs; for mild to moderate cases consider hypertonic oral solutions (broth) at iv NS.
- Pts will suddenly diuresis signaling a recovery for the inappropriate AVP secretion.
- If in a field environment consider transportation of all cases with sodium <130 or more severe symptoms (J Emerg Med 2001;21:47).
- Prevention strategies focus on limiting overhydration. Athletes in endurance events should consume fluids when thirsty and no more than 400-800 cc/hr (10-20 oz/hr) (Clin J Sp Med 2003;13:309).

21.4 Exercise-Induced Hematuria

Am Fam Phys 1996;53:905; Am Fam Phys 2005;71:6; Urol Clin N Am 1998;25:661; Adol Med 2003;14:3

Cause: Exercise.

Epidem: 15-30% of runners (specifically long-distance runners); 11-100% of all athletes.

Pathophys:
- Renal causes: jostling and shaking of the kidney, direct blow to kidney, increased glomerular permeability to RBC, or vasoconstriction and hypoxic damage to nephron.
- Bladder causes: repetitive impacts of the posterior vesicle wall against its base.
- Prostatic and urethral causes: direct trauma, esp in cyclists.

Sx: Usually none; may have discolored urine.

Si: Gross or microscopic hematuria.

Crs: Resolves with 24-72 hr of rest.

Cmplc: UTI, anemia.

Diff Dx: UTI/cystitis; upper tract disease; nephrolithiasis; STD; tumor; drugs/medications; dye ingestion.

Lab: UA, C&S, serum creatinine, urine cytology.

X-ray: Consider IVP.

Rx:
- Adequate hydration, and keep urine in bladder with running.
- Exercise moderation.
- Refer for >40 y/o, gross hematuria, recurrent sx, hematuria w no exercise or low intensity, and hematuria that does not clear w rest.

OTHER MEDICAL PROBLEMS

21.5 Exercise-Induced Asthma/Bronchospasm (AKA EIB or EIA)

Phy Sportsmed 1999;27:75; Clin Sports Med 1998;17:344; J Allergy Clin Imm 1998;101:646; Am Fam Phys 2003;67:4; Ped Clin North Am 2003;50:3

Cause:
- Vigorous physical activity.
- Cold, dry air especially asthmogenic.
- Tobacco smoke, sulfur dioxide, smog, molds, and pollens can aggravate.

Epidem: Occurs in up to 90% of individuals with chronic asthma and in 40% of those who have allergic rhinitis or atopic dermatitis; prevalence varies by sport; may be seen in 10-20% of competitive athletes.

Pathophys: Unknown, however there are two main theories:
1. Water Loss Theory: Normally, dry air is conditioned while passing through the nose, pharynx, and first seven generations of bronchi; w exercise, the ventilation rate increases and most breathing occurs through the mouth, bypassing conditioning; the airways become dry with alterations in osmolarity, pH, and temperature of the periciliary fluid; this results in mediator release and bronchoconstriction.
2. Heat Exchange Theory: Increased ventilation cools the airways during vigorous exercise; w the cessation of exercise; the bronchial vasculature dilates and engorges to rewarm the epithelium; engorged vessels then narrow the airways and may leak, resulting in mediator release and bronchospasm.

Sx:
- Shortness of breath, cough, wheezing, excessive sputum production, dyspnea, and/or chest tightness following 6-8 min of strenuous exercise.

- Avoidance of exercise in children.
- Inability to keep up w peers.
- Upset stomach or stomachache.
- Sore throat.
- Poorer performance than training predicts.

Si: Office exam may be normal or wheezing in chronic asthmatic pts.

Crs:

- Symptoms typically develop after 6-8 min of exercise at greater than 80% of maximum predicted HR.
- The greatest decrease in pulmonary function is seen about 15 min after exercise begins.
- Normal lung function returns 30-60 min after cessation of exercise.
- In about 30% of pts, particularly children, a late phase or second decrease in lung function may occur 6-8 hr after onset of exercise.
- 40-50% of pts with exercise-induced asthma may have a refractory period where exercise within 1-4 hr of initial activity does not induce symptoms.

Cmplc: Untreated, it may result in respiratory distress; decreased physical fitness, possibly poor self-image, poor peer-group acceptance as a result of avoiding regular childhood activities.

Diff Dx: Bronchitis, pneumonia, croup, CHF, congenital heart disease, hyperventilation, cystic fibrosis, pulmonary embolism, GERD, anaphylactic reaction, bronchopulmonary dysplasia, foreign body aspiration, laryngeal webs, chemical irritation, lymphadenopathy, vascular rings, tumor, laryngeal dysfunction.

Lab:

- Peak expiratory flow rate may be helpful during real-life event.
- Exercise challenge in a lab is most precise method of making diagnosis:

OTHER MEDICAL PROBLEMS

- Resting FEV_1 80-100% predicted; <80% predicted is indicative of chronic asthma.
- 5-8 min of high-intensity exercise (75-80% of maximum predicted HR) without warm-up.
- Spirometry is performed every 3 min following exercise and EIA is classified as mild, 15-20% drop in FEV_1, or severe, >30% drop in FEV_1.
- Metacholine challenge test may be useful if exercise testing is not conclusive; it is more sens but less spec than exercise testing.

Rx: Goal of management is to enable exercise at all intensity levels without respiratory limitations.

Nonpharmacologic:
- Exercise conditioning.
- Avoid exercise in cold, dry air.
- Avoid triggers and known triggering exercises.
- Cover nose and mouth w a scarf or breathing mask to warm and humidify air.
- Appropriate warm-up may induce refractory period.
- Cool down following activity.

Pharmacologic:
- Short-acting β_2-agonists 30 min prior to exercise provides prevention in up to 90% of cases; also used for treatment of acute symptoms (albuterol, terbutaline).
- Long-acting β_2-agonists 4 hr prior to exercise (salmeterol).
- Mast cell stabilizers 20 min prior to exercise may prevent symptoms in 70-80% of pts and have no side effects; may be effective in preventing late-phase symptoms (Intal, Tilade).
- Inhaled corticosteroids are helpful in pts with chronic asthma.
- Leukotriene modifiers may be effective in some cases (Accolate 20 mg po bid, Singulair 10 mg po qhs).
- Theophylline may be considered if there is inadequate response to standard prophylaxis.

NB: The USOC has banned all β_2-agonists except albuterol, terbutaline, and salmeterol.

21.6 Exercise-Induced Anaphylaxis

Phy Sportsmed 1996;24:76; Allergy: Principles and Practice. 5th ed. St. Louis: Mosby 1998;1109; Prim Care 1998;25:809; Clin Sports Med 1997;16:635; Immunol Aller Clin N Am 2004;24

Cause: Exercise is only trigger; in some individuals there is an associated food, such as celery, carrots, or wheat (food-dependent, exercise-induced anaphylaxis).

Epidem: Rare condition; more common in young people (mean 25 yrs); F:M ratio is 2:1; ²/₃ of pts have a family history of atopy and 50% are themselves atopic.

Pathophys: IgE-mediated release of mast cell products leading to smooth muscle spasm, bronchospasm, mucosal edema and inflammation, and increased capillary permeability.

Sx: Flushing sensation, pruritis, gi complaints such as vomiting, throat tightness or choking, headache.

Si: Diffuse, large urticarial wheals (10-25 mm), angioedema, bronchospasm, syncope, hypotension.

Crs:
- Symptoms typically begin soon after the start of exercise and resolve 30 min to 4 hr after cessation of activity.
- Attacks do not occur with every exercise session.
- Attacks are more common following meals in warm or humid environments (Phy Sportsmed 1996;24:76).

Cmplc: Untreated cases may progress to shock and airway obstruction, and are potentially life threatening.

Diff Dx: Physical urticarias, exercise-induced anaphylaxis variant syndrome, cholinergic urticaria.

Lab:
- Diagnosis is made from clinical history.

   NB: **Laboratory tests are expensive and nonspecific making them rarely helpful.**
- Exercise challenge tests are nonspec, and can be risky.

Rx:
- Acute treatment consists of immediate cessation of activity, movement to a cool place, and administration of injectable diphenhydramine.
- In pts with symptoms of throat tightness, dyspnea, and light-headedness, injectable epinephrine should be administered.
- Prophylactic treatment has been largely unsuccessful and remains controversial.
- Antihistamines have been shown in a few studies to decrease symptoms related to histamine release and remain the prophylaxis of choice.
- Pt precautions: pts with exercise-induced anaphylaxis should wear a medical bracelet, carry epinephrine, never exercise alone, avoid known food precipitants prior to exercise, and exercise in cool time of day.

21.7 Cholinergic Urticaria

Phy Sportsmed 1996;24; Allergy: Principles and Practice. 5th ed. St. Louis: Mosby 1998;1109; Prim Care 1998;25:809; Immunol All Clin N Am 2004;24

Cause: Process that raises the core body temperature by 0.5°C to 1.5°C (0.9°F to 2.7°F); specifically bathing in hot water, ingestion of spicy or hot foods.

Epidem: Rare condition; most common in young people (2nd or 3rd decades); found in approximately 5% of all cases of chronic urticaria; M=F.

Pathophys: Not fully elucidated; thought to be IgE-mediated release of mast cell products.

Sx: Headache, palpitations, abdominal cramps, diarrhea, sweating, flushing, lacrimation, salivation.

Si: Small pruritic papules (1-4 mm) with surrounding macular erythema; may be preceded by tingling, itching, or burning sensation of skin. Bronchospasm, hypotension, and angioedema may occur in rare cases.

Crs: Signs and symptoms develop 2-30 min following precipitant and last from 20-90 min.
  • Lesions appear first on upper thorax and neck, but can spread distally to involve the entire body.
  • Hives can become confluent and resemble angioedema.

Complc: Bronchospasm (clinically significant alteration in pulmonary function is unusual), angioedema, small risk of anaphylaxis, decreased fitness.

Diff Dx: Physical urticarias, exercise-induced anaphylaxis, exercise-induced anaphylaxis variant syndrome.

Lab:
  • Diagnosis made primarily by clinical history; laboratory tests are not helpful.
  • Warming an extremity to raise core temperature by 0.5-1.50°C is the most spec test.
  • Metacholine challenge test has only 50% sens.

Rx:
  • Avoid known triggers.
  • Hydroxyzine hydrochloride is the antihistamine of choice for prophylaxis; doses of 100 mg to 200 mg/24 hr divided qid are usually sufficient.
  • Diphenhydramine or hydroxyzine may be used for treatment at time of flare-up.
  • Epinephrine may be prescribed due to small risk of anaphylaxis.

OTHER MEDICAL PROBLEMS

Chapter 22

Basic Rehabilitation Exercises

22.1 Shoulder

Range of Motion

Figure 22.1 Pendulum exercises: Have pt bend forward at the waist with the upper trunk supported by the unaffected arm resting on a low table or chair; rotate the affected shoulder in slowly enlarging circles to improve range of motion.

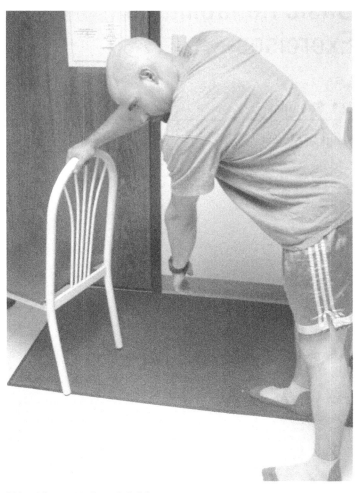

Figure 22.2 Wall climbs: Have pt stand at arms' length from a wall w the affected shoulder closer to the wall; abduct the arm as far as possible; if abduction not full, then complete full abduction by climbing up the wall w the fingers; the pt may need to step closer to the wall as abducting. Repeat 5 × per session, 3 sessions per d.

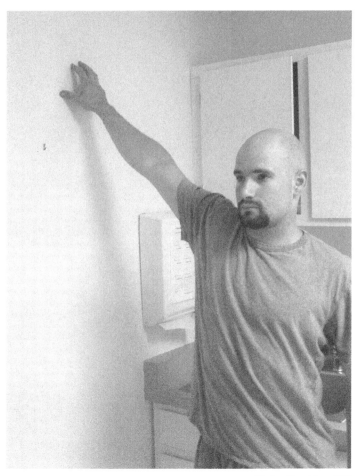

Figure 22.3 Posterior capsular stretch: Adduct affected arm across chest. Use opposite arm to further adduct, stretching the posterior capsule of the affected arm. Hold for 10-15 sec; 5 × per session, 2-3 sessions per d.

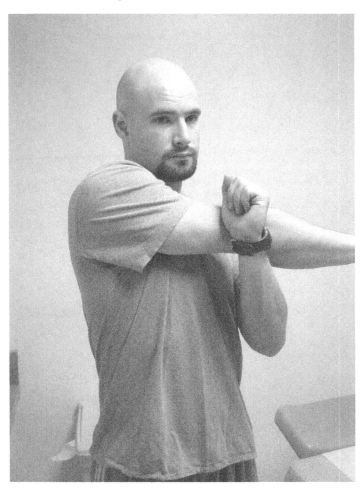

Figure 22.4 Towel stretch: Place affected arm on sacrum. W a towel and the opposite arm further stretch the affected arm by pulling upward. Hold for 10-15 sec; 5 reps per session, 3 sessions per d.

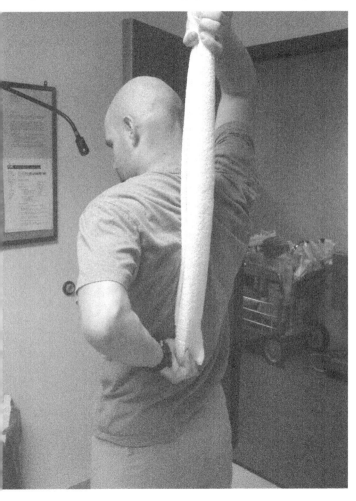

Strengthening

Figure 22.5 Supraspinatus: Have pt abduct arm w thumb pointed down to 60°; use free-wts (3-5 lb). Hold for 5 sec; 12-15 reps per set and 3 sets per d.

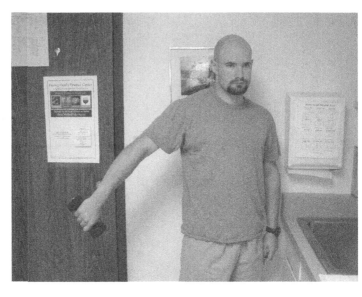

Figure 22.6 External rotators: Pt lying on side externally rotates lifting a 3-5 lb wt to parallel and holds for 5 sec. Perform 12-15 reps per session and 3 sets/d.

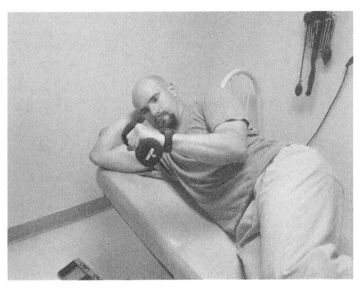

Internal rotation: While lying on side as with external rotators, have pt place wt in lower arm and rotator toward the chest (internal rotation), lifting a 3-5 lb wt and hold for 5 sec; perform 12-15 reps per session; 3 sessions per d.

Figure 22.7 Scapular stabilizers: From prone position, w head on rolled towel and 3-5 lb wts in each arm, have pt pull scapulae together lifting the wt off the ground. Hold for 5 sec; perform 10-15 reps, 3 sessions per d.

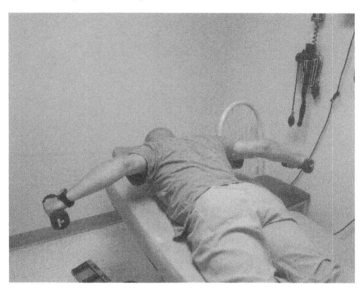

22.2 Elbow

Stretching

Figure 22.8 Flexors: Have pt extend elbow and wrist and max supination. Hold for 10-15 sec, 5 reps per session and 3 sessions per d.

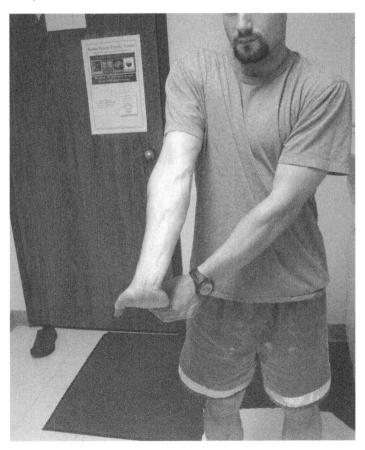

Figure 22.9 Extensors: Have pt extend elbow and flex wrist w max pronation. Hold for 10-15 sec; 5 reps per session, 3 sessions per d.

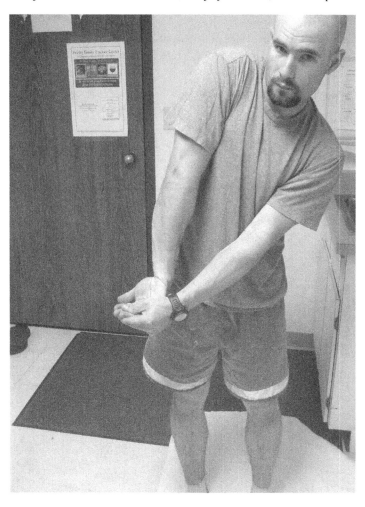

Strengthening

Figure 22.10 Flexors: W elbow and forearm resting on thigh w 3-5 lb
wt in hand, have pt flex the wrist and hold for 5 sec, then lower
to a 3 count; perform 10-15 reps, 3 sets per d.

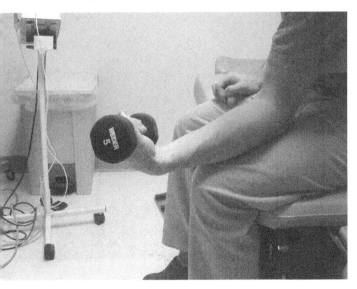

Figure 22.11 Extensors: W elbow and forearm resting on thigh w 3-5 lb wt in hand, have pt extend wrist and hold for 5 sec, then lower to a 3 count; perform 10-15 reps and 3 sets per day.

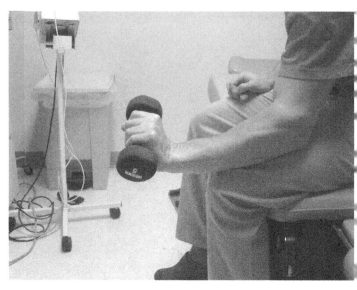

Figure 22.12 Rope exercises: Tie a 5 lb free-wt on a rope to an old broomstick. Hold arms out in front of the body and roll the broomstick elevating the wt to the stick then lower slowly. Start with 5 reps per session working up to 10-15 reps and 3 sessions per d.

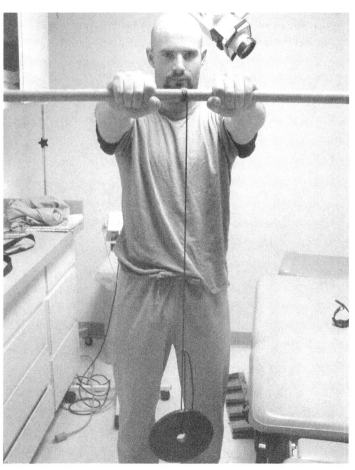

22.3 Back

Stretching/ROM

Knee chest stretch:

Figure 22.13 Single leg: Have pt slowly pull the bent knee toward opposite shoulder, while keeping the other knee and lower back against the floor.

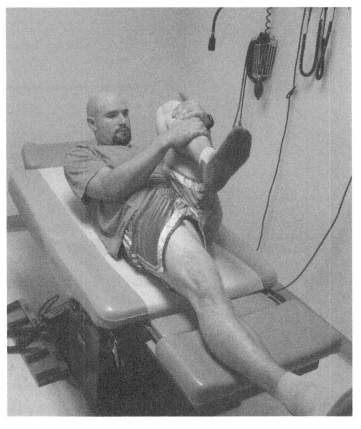

Figure 22.14 Double leg: Have pt gently pull both knees to the chest; hold for 15 sec and repeat 5 × per session and 3 sessions per d

If ROM not full due to pain, have pt pull w each exercise to the point of pain, and then attempt to straighten either a single or double knees against clasped hands for a count of 10, then relax and pull closer to the chest and repeat.

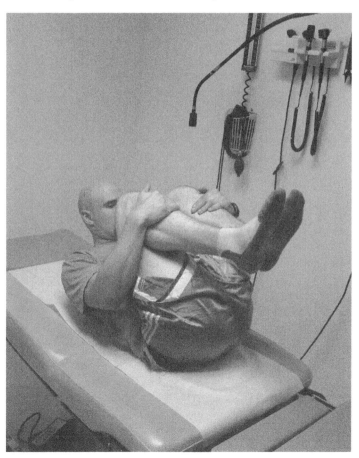

Figure 22.15 Hamstring stretch: Have pt lie on back and bring one knee up toward the chest; thigh is supported in the vertical position; pt then slowly straightens the knee by contracting the quads, and stretches the hamstrings; holds for 15-20 sec, repeats 5 ×, 3 sessions per d.

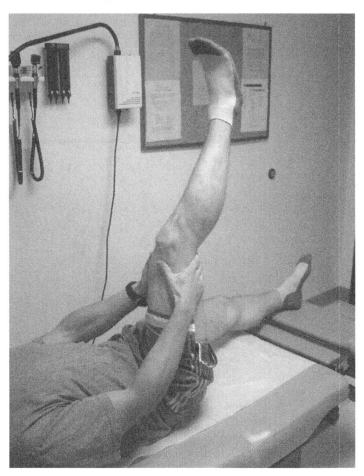

Figure 22.16 Hip flexor stretch: Have pt place hands on hips in a one-legged kneeling position; keeping the abdominal muscles tight slowly lunges forward, stretching the hip flexors of the kneeling leg.

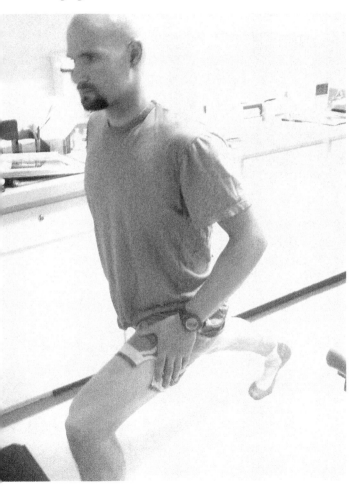

Figure 22.17 Piriformis stretch: While sitting in chair and affected leg crossed with ankle resting on opposite knee, pt rotates chest toward the knee of the crossed leg and forward bends at the waist, keeping the back straight as if pushing the sternum to the knee. Hold for 10-15 sec; 5 reps per session, 3 sessions per d.

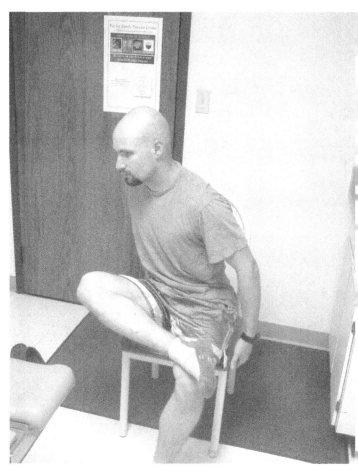

Strengthening The Core

Figure 22.18 Crunches: Have pt fold arms across chest in sit-up position, forward flex at the waist until the scapulae are off the floor. Hold for 5 sec; repeat 10-15 ×, 3 sessions per d.

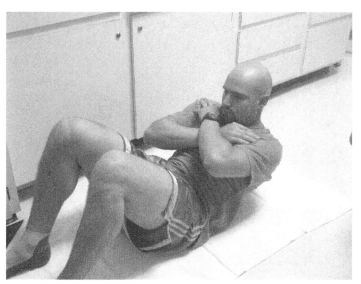

Figure 22.19 Pelvic tilt: Have pt tighten the abdomen pressing the lower back to the floor and tilting the symphysis toward the head; hold for 5-10 sec; repeat 10 × and 3 sessions per d.

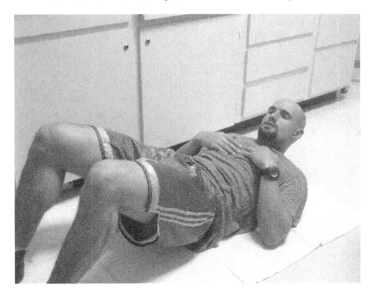

Figure 22.20 Back bridge: Have pt resting on back with arms on floor and legs bent 90°. Raise the buttocks in the air until the back is straight. Hold for 10-15 sec; 10 reps per session and 3 sessions per d.

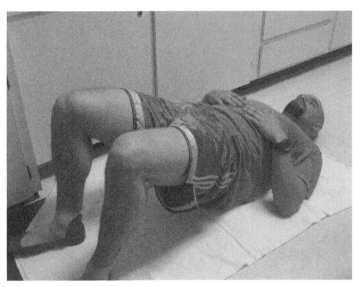

Figure 22.21 Opposite arm and leg: While on all fours, have pt extend the opposite arm and leg maximally and hold for 10 sec; perform 10 reps per session, 3 sessions per d.

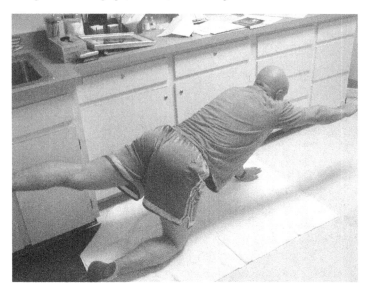

Figure 22.22 Side lifts: While resting on elbow on side lift the hips off the floor; have pt make the body straight and hold for 10 sec; repeat 10-15 ×, 3 sessions per d.

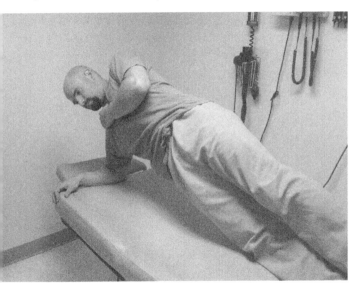

22.4 Knee

Stretching

Figure 22.23 ITB: Pt leans against a wall or pole w arm straight and drives hip toward the wall. Hips perpendicular to wall. Step over for balance only. Hold for 15-20 sec, 5 reps per session, 3 sessions per d.

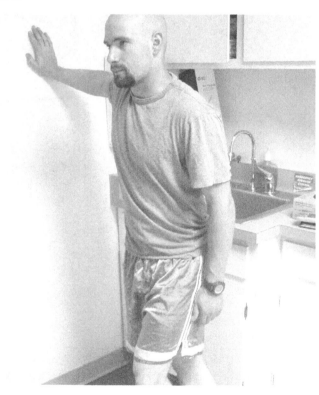

Hamstrings: See figure 22.15.

Hip flexors: See figure 22.16.

Figure 22.24 Quads: Pt leans against a wall w heel in buttock; held w the opposite hand; stand erect on the single leg and straighten or extend hip to stretch the quads; hold for 15 sec, repeat 5-10 ×, 3 sessions per d.

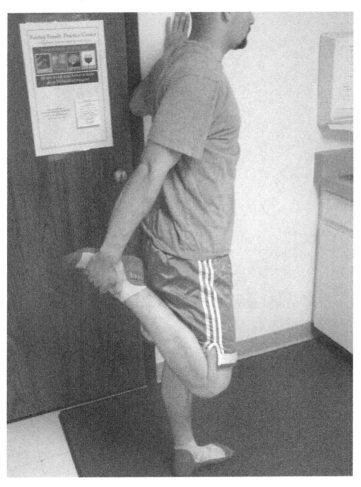

Strengthening

Figure 22.25 Hip abductor strengthening: Lying on side, have pt abduct the top leg 40-45° and hold for 10 sec. Repeat 15-20 reps 3 sessions per d. When this is easily accomplished, add a 1-lb ankle wt.

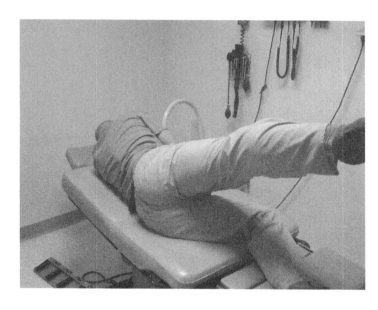

Figure 22.26 Quad sets: In seated or partially reclined position with a rolled towel supporting the knee, have pt tighten the quads and raise the leg 6-12 inches off the surface of the floor and hold for 5-10 sec, repeat 10-15 ×, 3 sessions per d.

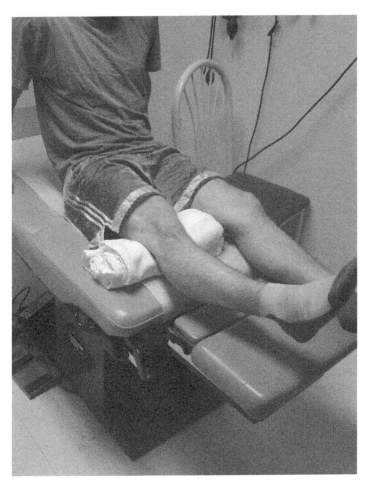

Figure 22.27 Muncie technique: Pt sits on flat surface w affected leg straight and opposite leg flexed. Pt leans toward the bent knee, rotates the straight leg out, locks the knee, raises 1 inch, holds for 5 sec, then rests. Repeat 20 × each d. Made harder by bending forward at the waist toward the bent knee.

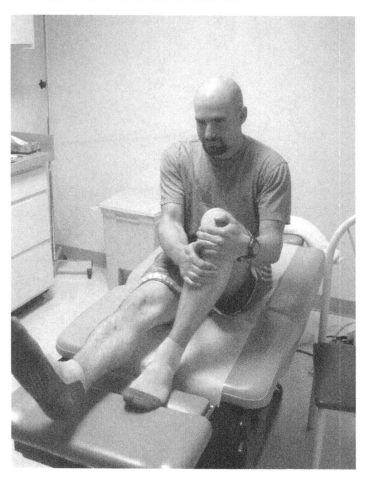

Figure 22.28 Wall sits: Have pt stand with legs shoulder width apart and about 12-18 inches from a wall or door with back on wall. Squat about 30-40° and hold for 15 sec, repeat 10-15 ×, 3 sessions per d.

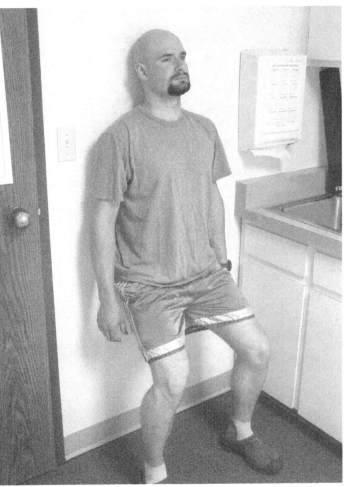

Figure 22.29 Stair dips: Pt stands on stair with one leg on stair and one hanging while facing one wall. Bending the "standing knee," pt slowly lowers self keeping back straight and hips level until lower (hanging) foot touches lower step. Pt rises slowly to starting position. Repeat slowly 10-15 reps 3 sessions per d.

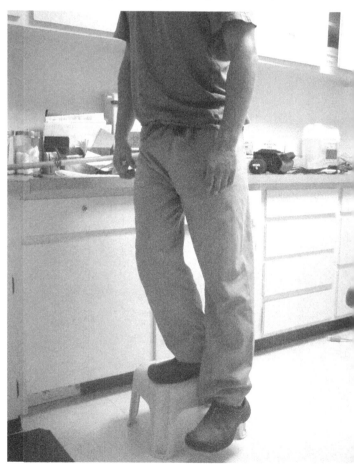

22.5 Ankle

Stretching

Figure 22.30 Achilles: Have pt place the injured foot behind the un-injured foot and keep the back knee straight w the heel firmly planted on the ground; lean forward against the wall, while keeping the back foot pointed straight; hold for 20-25 sec, repeat 5-10 ×, 3 sessions per d.

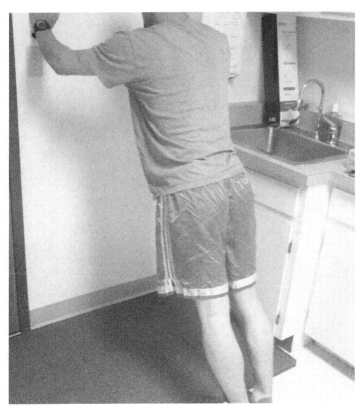

Strengthening (isometric)

Figure 22.31 Peroneal isometrics: Have pt stand or sit and place the outside of the injured foot against a door jamb; pushes outward w the foot for 5-10 sec, repeat 10 ×, 3 sessions per d.

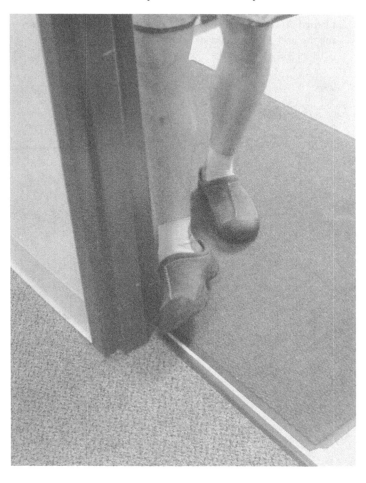

Figure 22.32 Posterior tibialis isometric: Have pt stand or sit and place the inside of the injured foot against a door jamb; push inward w the foot for 5-10 sec, repeat 10 ×, 3 sessions per d.

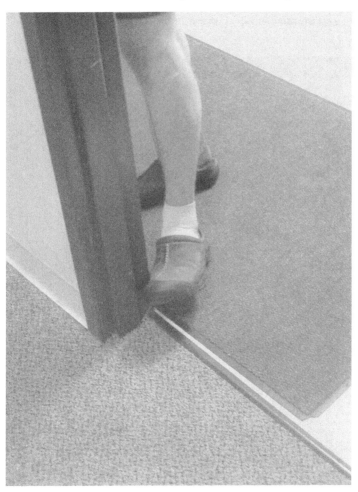

Figure 22.33 Single leg balance (proprioceptive drill): Have pt stand on the affected leg on a firm surface (concrete, hardwood, tile) w eyes open for 30-60 sec. When this is mastered, attempt the same drill with eyes closed, and then standing on a folded hand towel on the same surface. Perform 10 reps/session and 3 sessions/d.

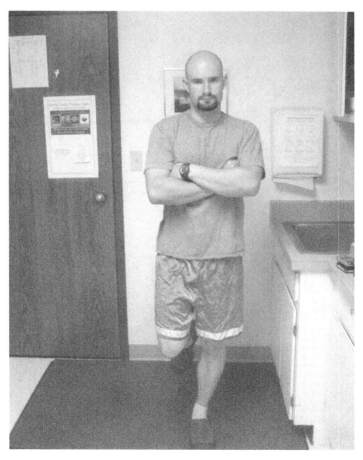

Index

Neck strain. *See* cervical sprain
Neer impingement sign, 85
Neuropsychometric testing, for
    concussions, 272
Nutrition. *See also* eating disorders, in
    female athletes
    guidelines for optimum
        performance, 41
    U.S. government guidelines for, 41

O

Ober's test, 178
    for greater trochanter bursitis, 178
    for Iliotibial band friction
        syndrome, 213
Obrien test for SLAP lesions, 94
Olecranon bursitis, 104
Os trigonum syndrome, 265
Osborne wave in hypothermia, 33
Osgood-Schlatter disease (OSD), 294
    Sinding-Larsen-Johanssen vs., 295
Osteitis pubis, 176
Osteoarthritis
    acromioclavicular, 79
    rotator cuff tear vs., 75
    tendinosis vs., 89
Osteochondral defect (OCD) of the
    talus, 237
Osteochondritis dessicans (OCD)
    of the elbow, 291
    of the knee, 289
Osteoid osteoma, vs.
    acromioclavicular osteoarthritis,
    80
Osteoporosis, in female athletes, 327
Overtraining, 351
    differential diagnosis, 353
    evaluation of, 353
    hypotheses, 351–352

P

Palmer space infection, 133
Pancreatitis, vs. mechanical low back
    pain, 156
Panner's disease, 291
Pars interarticularis, 283
Patellar apprehension test, 197
Patellar dislocation, 196
    ACL injury vs., 189
    posterior cruciate injury vs., 192
Patellar grind test, 205
Patellar subluxation, 196
Patellar tendinitis, 206
    Osgood-Schlatter disease vs., 294
    patellofemoral pain vs., 204
Patellar tendon rupture, 199
Patellofemoral pain, 204
Pendulum exercises for shoulder
    injuries, 366
Periostalgia. *See* medial tibial stress
    syndrome
Peritendonitis, vs. Achilles
    tendinopathy, 248
Pernio. *See* chilblains
Peroneal tendon subluxation, 233
Pes anserine bursitis, 210
Phalangeal fractures
    foot, 256
    hand, middle, 121
    hand, proximal, 123
Phalen's test, for carpal tunnel
    syndrome, 277
Pheochromocytoma, vs. stimulants, 49
PIP fracture dislocation, 122
PIP volar plate rupture, 118
Piriformis syndrome, 181
    discogenic back pain vs., 158
Pitcher's elbow. *See* medial
    epicondylitis
Pivot shift test for ACL tear, 190

Made in the USA
Las Vegas, NV
10 July 2022